3D Printing: Applications in Medicine and Surgery

3D Printing: Applications in Medicine and Surgery

Volume 1

Edited by

Georgios Tsoulfas, MD, PhD

Associate Professor of Surgery
Aristotle University of Thessaloniki
Thessaloniki, Greece

Petros I. Bangeas

General Surgeon
Academic Scholar
First Department of Surgery
Aristotle University of Thessaloniki
Thessaloniki, Greece

Jasjit S. Suri, PhD, MBA, FAIMBE, FAIUM

Global Biomedical Technologies, Inc.,
California, United States

ELSEVIER

Elsevier
Radarweg 29, PO Box 211, 1000 AE Amsterdam, Netherlands
The Boulevard, Langford Lane, Kidlington, Oxford OX5 1GB, United Kingdom
50 Hampshire Street, 5th Floor, Cambridge, MA 02139, United States

Notices

Practitioners and researchers must always rely on their own experience and knowledge in evaluating and using any information, methods, compounds or experiments described herein. Because of rapid advances in the medical sciences, in particular, independent verification of diagnoses and drug dosages should be made. To the fullest extent of the law, no responsibility is assumed by Elsevier, authors, editors or contributors for any injury and/or damage to persons or property as a matter of products liability, negligence or otherwise, or from any use or operation of any methods, products, instructions, or ideas contained in the material herein.

ISBN: 978-0-323-66164-5

Publisher: Cathleen Sether
Acquisition Editor: Jessica McCool
Editorial Project Manager: Samantha Allard
Production Project Manager: Kiruthika Govindaraju
Cover Designer: Alan Studholme

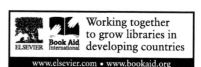

Working together
to grow libraries in
developing countries

www.elsevier.com • www.bookaid.org

Contents

Contributors

Kyriakos Anastasiadis, MD, PhD, FETCS, FCCP
Department of Cardiothoracic Surgery, Aristotle University of Thessaloniki, AHEPA University Hospital, Thessaloniki, Greece

Elissavet Anestiadou
Medical Department, Aristotle University of Thessaloniki, Thessaloniki, Greece

Petros I. Bangeas
General Surgeon, Academic Scholar, First Department of Surgery, Aristotle University of Thessaloniki, Thessaloniki, Greece

Vasiliki Bisbinas
Medical Department, Aristotle University of Thessaloniki, Thessaloniki, Greece

Jannis Constantinidis
ENT Department, Aristotle University of Thessaloniki, AHEPA Hospital, Thessaloniki, Greece

Ioannis Dagkinis, PhD
Department of Shipping Trade & Transport, University of the Aegean, Chios, Greece

Efstratios Georgakarakos, MD, MSc, PhD
Assistant Professor of Vascular Surgery, Department of Vascular Surgery, Medical School, University Hospital of Alexandroupolis, Democritus University of Thrace, Alexandroupolis, Greece

Georgios Georgantis, MD, PhD
Academic Fellow, Aristotle University of Thessaloniki, Thessaloniki, Greece

Petros D. Karkos
ENT Department, Aristotle University of Thessaloniki, AHEPA Hospital, Thessaloniki, Greece

Ion-Anastasios Karolos, PhD
Rural and Surveying Engineer, School of Rural and Surveying Engineering, Aristotle University of Thessaloniki, Thessaloniki, Greece

Eustathios Kenanidis, MD, PhD, MSc
Academic Orthopaedic Department, Papageorgiou General Hospital, Aristotle University Medical School, Thessaloniki, Greece; Center of Orthopaedic and Regenerative Medicine (C.O.RE.) - Center for Interdisciplinary Research and Innovation — Aristotle University Thessaloniki (C.I.R.I.-AU.Th), Balkan Center, Buildings A & B, Thessaloniki, Greece

Evanthia Kostidi, PhD
Department of Shipping Trade & Transport, University of the Aegean, Chios, Greece

Georgios Koufopoulos, MD
Medical School, Democritus University of Thrace, Alexandroupolis, Greece

Georgios Lales
Medical Department, Aristotle University of Thessaloniki, Thessaloniki, Greece

Charles M. Miller, MD
Department of Hepato-Pancreato-Biliary and Transplant Surgery, Digestive Disease Institute, Cleveland Clinic, Cleveland, OH, United States; Enterprise Director of Transplantation, Transplantation Center, Digestive Disease and Surgery Institute, Cleveland, OH, United States

Nikitas Nikitakos
Professor, Department of Shipping Trade & Transport, University of the Aegean, Chios, Greece

Dimitrios Papachristos, PhD
University of West Attica, Greece

Vasileios N. Papadopoulos
Professor of Surgery and Chairman of the First Department of Surgery, Aristotle University of Thessaloniki School of Medicine, Thessaloniki, Greece

Christos Pikridas, PhD
Professor, Rural and Surveying Engineer, School of Rural and Surveying Engineering, Department of Geodesy and Surveying, Aristotle University of Thessaloniki, Thessaloniki, Greece

Michael Potoupnis, MD, PhD
Academic Orthopaedic Department, Papageorgiou General Hospital, Aristotle University Medical School, Thessaloniki, Greece; Center of Orthopaedic and Regenerative Medicine (C.O.RE.) - Center for Interdisciplinary Research and Innovation — Aristotle University Thessaloniki (C.I.R.I.-AU.Th), Balkan Center, Buildings A & B, Thessaloniki, Greece

Cristiano Quintini, MD
Department of Hepato-Pancreato-Biliary and Transplant Surgery, Digestive Disease Institute, Cleveland Clinic, Cleveland, OH, United States; Director, Associate Professor of Surgery, Cleveland Clinic Lerner College of Medicine, Liver Tranpslantation, General Surgery, Cleveland Clinic, Cleveland, OH, United States

Konstantinos Skarentzos, MS
Medical School, Democritus University of Thrace, Alexandroupolis, Greece

Marios Stavrakas
ENT Department, Aristotle University of Thessaloniki, AHEPA Hospital, Thessaloniki, Greece

Jasjit S. Suri, PhD, MBA, FAIMBE, FAIUM
Global Biomedical Technologies, Inc., California, United States

Georgios I. Tagarakis, MD, PhD, FETCS
Department of Cardiothoracic Surgery, Aristotle University of Thessaloniki,
AHEPA University Hospital, Thessaloniki, Greece

Vassilios Tsioukas, PhD
Electrical Engineer, Professor, School of Rural and Surveying Engineering,
Aristotle University of Thessaloniki, Thessaloniki, Greece

Eleftherios Tsiridis, MD, MSc, PhD, FACS, FRCS
Academic Orthopaedic Department, Papageorgiou General Hospital, Aristotle
University Medical School, Thessaloniki, Greece; Center of Orthopaedic and
Regenerative Medicine (C.O.RE.) - Center for Interdisciplinary Research and
Innovation – Aristotle University Thessaloniki (C.I.R.I.-AU.Th), Balkan Center,
Buildings A & B, Thessaloniki, Greece

Georgios Tsoulfas, MD, PhD
Associate Professor, Department of Surgery, Aristotle University of Thessaloniki,
Thessaloniki, Greece

Anastasios-Nektarios Tzavellas, MD, MSc
Academic Orthopaedic Department, Papageorgiou General Hospital, Aristotle
University Medical School, Thessaloniki, Greece; Center of Orthopaedic and
Regenerative Medicine (C.O.RE.) - Center for Interdisciplinary Research and
Innovation – Aristotle University Thessaloniki (C.I.R.I.-AU.Th), Balkan Center,
Buildings A & B, Thessaloniki, Greece; Orthopaedic Surgeon, 2nd Department of
Orthopaedic and Trauma Surgery, 424 Military General Hospital, Thessaloniki,
Greece

Takis Vidalis, PhD
Senior Scientist, Legal Advisor, Hellenic National Bioethics Commission, Attica,
Greece

Nizar N. Zein, MD
Department of Gastroenterology and Hepatology, Digestive Disease Institute,
Cleveland Clinic, Cleveland, OH, United States; Director, Mikati Liver Center,
Digestive Disease and Surgery Institute, The Cleveland Clinic, Cleveland, OH,
United States; Chair, Global Patient Services, The Cleveland Clinic, Cleveland,
OH, United States

Ioannis A. Ziogas, MD
First Department of Surgery, Aristotle University of Thessaloniki, Thessaloniki,
Greece; Postdoctoral Research Fellow, Division of Hepatobiliary Surgery and Liver
Transplantation, Section of Surgical Sciences, Vanderbilt University Medical
Center, Nashville, TN, United States

Introduction: the role of 3D printing in surgery

1

Georgios Tsoulfas, MD, PhD[1], Petros I. Bangeas[2],
Jasjit S. Suri, PhD, MBA, FAIMBE, FAIUM[3], Vasileios N. Papadopoulos[4]

[1]*Associate Professor, Department of Surgery, Aristotle University of Thessaloniki, Thessaloniki, Greece;* [2]*General Surgeon, Academic Scholar, First Department of Surgery, Aristotle University of Thessaloniki, Thessaloniki, Greece;* [3]*Global Biomedical Technologies, Inc., California, United States;* [4]*Professor of Surgery and Chairman of the First Department of Surgery, Aristotle University of Thessaloniki School of Medicine, Thessaloniki, Greece*

Introduction

The last few decades have seen tremendous progress in surgery with the incorporation of several technological advancements, leading to the increased practice of minimally invasive surgical procedures in general surgery and all the different surgical specialties and subspecialties. The overall goal has been to achieve a more targeted, patient-oriented approach which would combine curing the patient, while at the same time preserving quality and safety of care. One of the more recent technological developments that has left a significant imprint in industry with product design and manufacturing and aeronautics is 3D printing [1]. The amazing success and wide-spread applications of 3D printing meant that it was only a matter of time till this technology drew the interest of physicians and surgeons, interested in expanding these applications in medicine and surgery [2]. Similar to the advent of any new technology and especially in the age of the internet and social media, this led initially to a situation where science and science fiction played equal parts in trying to explain this new technology and its applications; before we could print basic instruments, we would hear talk about 3D printing of human organs. This is not necessarily wrong, as before you create something new, you need to dream of it first before facing the practical realities of realizing your goals. However, it is our duty to stay grounded and ensure that any new technology and its applications in any field, and much more so when it pertains to human lives, are carefully and fully evaluated.

The technology of 3D printing, together with areas such as nanotechnology and biomedicine, are all part of the regenerative medicine effort. This represents a field where engineering and medicine come together to identify ways of preserving or, more likely, replacing basic biological functions in an effort to sustain and improve life. This is a core part of surgery, as it can provide us with answers and solutions to many of the problems that surgeons have to face, including organ failure due to trauma, infection, cancer, or even the frailty of age. This becomes even more critical if we consider the increased longevity of the population together with the increased

3D Printing: Applications in Medicine and Surgery. https://doi.org/10.1016/B978-0-323-66164-5.00001-5

expectations. Before embarking on this quest, however, it is imperative that certain questions are answered, including

- The history and current status of 3D printing
- What are the possible applications of 3D printing in surgery today?
- What are the challenges and future prospects for 3D printing in surgery?

This chapter will provide a brief overview of the topic and these questions, with the main part to follow in the rest of the book.

History of 3D printing

In the early part of the 1990s, we witnessed the first laboratory arrangements of stereo-lithography, which eventually led to the automated natural prototype production, through a process of layering of resin levels that were solidified with the use of a laser. This process had originally received an intellectual property patent in 1986 by Charles Hull, and in 1987, the first machine was presented by 3D Systems Inc [3]. The concept is based on a process of additive layering of the material to create the 3D object. Similar to the inkjet printer concept, in 3D printing there is the initial additive layering of a polymer (or any material that can reach liquid stage through heat) which is placed horizontally and then solidified either through cooling or through ultraviolet radiation, so that a complete 3D model can be printed. Every horizontal layer is similar to the pictures obtained during a computed tomography scan (CT scan) or any similar radio-logical two-dimensional picture. The challenge is converting the data from these two-dimensional representations through the use of stereolithography to an .stl file that can be used to obtain the 3D-printed product. This was originally used in the industry as a way to design and manufacture new products, with the main advantage of the 3D printer being the speed compared to more traditional methods.

At the same time, this basic description of the process also reveals some of the main limitations or challenges. Specifically, the final product is only as good as the original design of what will be printed; that is in order, for example, to 3D print an organ based on a CT scan, it is critical that both the CT scan and the method of information transmission to the 3D printer are as detailed as possible. Additionally, another challenge is the type of material used, the number of colors needed and other manufacturing issues, all of which increase the complexity of the 3D printer needed. Not surprisingly this has direct bearing on the cost of the whole process, as 3D printer prices can range from several hundred to several hundred thousand US dollars. The speed of the printer, the ability to use different materials, and the layering method used are some of the more important factors explaining the differences in cost.

3D printing in surgery

One of the main advantages of 3D printing and the main reason for the introduction of 3D printing in surgery was the ability to convert 2D pictures into a 3D object. This enabled the surgeon to better understand the anatomy of the lesion and the surrounding area, thus being able to plan the surgery in a more efficient manner [2,4,5]. The ability to simulate an operation has been helpful to the whole surgical team, including residents, fellows, and students, which resulted in application of the 3D printing technology in surgical fields such as neurosurgery, cardiothoracic surgery, plastic surgery, facial reconstructive surgery, and orthopedic surgery [6,7]. It allowed surgeons to envision in a clear manner the complicated anatomy involving blood vessels, nerves, and surrounding bone structures, allowing for significantly fewer complications. Studies comparing the 3D-printed models to cadaveric ones for the purposes of planning and simulating a cardiac operation showed no difference, even with the earlier 3D-printed attempts [8,9]. The same was possible in other surgical specialties including liver transplantation, where it was possible to map the liver of a living donor and accurately assess the volume and the part of the liver required for the transplantation [10,11]. Similarly, 3D printing also played a key role in the transplantation of a kidney from an adult living donor to a pediatric recipient as it allowed the surgical team to simulate the anatomy and the placement of the renal graft in the recipient [12]. Being able to evaluate the exact hepatic volume and the blood and biliary vessels involved allowed for a more targeted approach in a surgery involving a living donor, which is an essential step in ensuring the safety of the living donor. In the case of the living renal transplantation, especially in a pediatric population, the improved simulation offered by 3D printing also means avoiding exploration on the surgical table and thus improved safety and decreased operative time. If we add to all of the above, the significantly reduced cost and regulatory burden of the 3D-printed models compared to the cadaveric ones, it is easy to understand the appeal of the new technology.

The next step in the evolution of the technology was the actual 3D printing of material to be used in the surgery, such as grafts for closure of skull defects or for orthopedic procedures, with applications in craniofacial surgery, neurosurgery, and orthopedic surgery [13–15]. The ability to 3D print a graft that would fit exactly the specific patient was crucial in avoiding future surgeries. Another factor was the complete lack of immunogenicity of the material used which led to decreased inflammation. An extension of the process of 3D printing of material to be used in a surgery was 3D printing of actual surgical instruments [16–18]. Together with the use of nanotechnology, this allowed for antibiotic coating of these instruments providing surgeons with an instrument to their exact specifications, which was also potentially safer for the patient. One of the implications of this technique and approach is its importance for global and humanitarian surgery, as the ability to 3D print inexpensive instruments in underdeveloped areas of the world (which also happen to be the ones with the greatest medical need) can affect the lives of millions of people.

Another application of 3D printing, in addition to helping simulate a surgery and printing material to be used during the surgery, is its role in patient and family education regarding the upcoming procedure. In order for the patients and their families to understand the surgery planned and the risks involved, so that they can provide informed consent, the ability to examine a 3D model of the relevant anatomy can be very helpful. The surgical team can better discuss the procedure and potential complications with the use of such a model and answer any relevant questions. There have been several studies confirming the importance of 3D-printed models in helping patients and their families understand the underlying pathology and the type of treatment planned [19–21].

Conclusion

The advent of 3D printing represents an excellent example of how technological advancements can potentially change surgical practice. In the short time period since the first applications, it has been possible to see the effect that it has had and continues to have allowing surgeons to simulate the operation planned, improving the education of surgical trainees and helping patients and their families better understand the upcoming surgery and the risks involved. This is potentially only the beginning, for as we are able to understand the technology and its limitations better new areas of clinical applications emerge, including the possibility of 3D organ and tissue printing with the use of bioprinting. However, before all of this is realized, we need to understand and overcome several obstacles, including the cost, the need for improved printing technology, better materials, and increased understanding of the technology. Critical factors are the need for interdisciplinary collaboration between surgeons and engineers, as well as an understanding that nature is much more complex than it first appears.

This book will provide readers with an overview of what is 3D printing and its applications in surgery, including an examination of its role in several surgical specialties and subspecialties. At the same time, as it is necessary with any new technology, ethical and organizational issues will be addressed in order to provide readers with a more complete picture of what the future holds.

References

[1] Artzi D, Kroll E. Enhancing aerospace engineering students' learning with 3D printing wind-tunnel models. Rapid Prototyp J 2011;17(5):393–402.
[2] Bangeas P. Contribution of Three Dimensional Printing in the Manufacturing of Surgical Materials With Antimicrobial Properties. Postgraduate study, Aristotle University of Thessaloniki; 2016.
[3] Charles H, Michael F, Yehudah B, Roy S, Emanuel S, Allan L, Terry W. Rapid prototyping: current technology and future potential. Rapid Prototyp J 1995;1(1):11–9.
[4] Biglino G, Verschueren P, Zegels R, Taylor AM, Schievano S. Rapid prototyping compliant arterial phantoms for in-vitro studies and device testing. J Cardiovasc Magn Reson 2013;15(1):2.

[5]   Martelli N, Serrano C, van den Brink H, Pineau J, Prognon P, Borget I, El Batti S. Advantages and disadvantages of 3-dimensional printing in surgery: a systematic review. Surgery 2016;159(6):1485−500.

[6]   Ayoub AF, Rehab M, O'Neil M, Khambay B, Ju X, Barbenel J, Naudi K. A novel approach for planning orthognathic surgery: the integration of dental casts into three-dimensional printed mandibular models. Int J Oral Maxillofac Surg 2014;43(4):454−9.

[7]   Sodian R, Schmauss D, Markert M, Weber S, Nikolaou K, Haeberle S, Vogt F, Vicol C, Lueth T, Reichart B, Schmitz C. Three-dimensional printing creates models for surgical planning of aortic valve replacement after previous coronary bypass grafting. Ann Thorac Surg 2008;85(6):2105−8.

[8]   Costello JP, Olivieri LJ, Krieger A, Thabit O, Marshall MB, Yoo SJ, Kim PC, Jonas RA, Nath DS. Utilizing three-dimensional printing technology to assess the feasibility of high-fidelity synthetic ventricular septal defect models for simulation in medical education. World J Pediatr Congenit Heart Surg 2014;5(3):421−6.

[9]   Bangeas P, Drevelegas K, Agorastou C, Tzounis L, Chorti A, Paramythiotis D, Michalopoulos A, Tsoulfas G, Papadopoulos VN, Exadaktylos A, Suri JS. Three-dimensional printing as an educational tool in colorectal surgery. Front Biosci 2019 Jan 1;11:29−37.

[10] Duan B, Kapetanovic E, Hockaday LA, Butcher JT. Three-dimensional printed trileaflet valve conduits using biological hydrogels and human valve interstitial cells. Acta Biomater 2014;10(5):1836−46.

[11] Zein NN, Hanouneh IA, Bishop PD, Samaan M, Eghtesad B, Quintini C, Miller C, Yerian L, Klatte R. Three-dimensional print of a liver for preoperative planning in living donor liver transplantation. Liver Transpl 2013;19(12):1304−10.

[12] Chandak P, Byrne N, Coleman A, Karunanithy N, Carmichael J, Marks SD, Stojanovic J, Kessaris N, Mamode N. Patient-specific 3D printing: a novel technique for complex pediatric renal transplantation. Ann Surg February 2019;269(2):e18−23.

[13] Skelley NW, Smith MJ, Ma R, Cook JL. Three-dimensional printing technology in orthopaedics. J Am Acad Orthop Surg July 1, 2019. https://doi.org/10.5435/JAAOS-D-18-00746 [Epub ahead of print] PMID: 31268868.

[14] Sultan AA, Mahmood B, Samuel LT, Stearns KL, Molloy RM, Moskal JT, Krebs VE, Harwin SF, Mont MA. Cementless 3D printed highly porous titanium-coated baseplate total knee arthroplasty: survivorship and outcomes at 2-year minimum follow-up. J Knee Surg February 6, 2019. https://doi.org/10.1055/s-0039-1677842 [Epub ahead of print].

[15] Luo J, Morrison DA, Hayes AJ, Bala A, Watts G. Single-piece titanium plate cranioplasty reconstruction of complex defects. J Craniofac Surg June 2018;29(4):839−42.

[16] Ballard DH, Tappa K, Boyer CJ, Jammalamadaka U, Hemmanur K, Weisman JA, Alexander JS, Mills DK, Woodard PK. Antibiotics in 3D-printed implants, instruments and materials: benefits, challenges and future directions. J 3D Print Med. June 2019; 3(2):83−93.

[17] Pakzaban P. A 3-dimensional-printed spine localizer: introducing the concept of online dissemination of novel surgical instruments. Neurospine September 2018;15(3):242−8.

[18] Weisman JA, Ballard DH, Jammalamadaka U, Tappa K, Sumerel J, D'Agostino HB, Mills DK, Woodard PK. 3D printed antibiotic and chemotherapeutic eluting catheters for potential use in interventional radiology: in vitro proof of concept study. Acad Radiol February 2019;26(2):270−4.

[19] Kim PS, Choi CH, Han IH, Lee JH, Choi HJ, Lee JI. Obtaining informed consent using patient specific 3D printing cerebral aneurysm model. J Korean Neurosurg Soc July 2019;62(4):398−404.

[20] Biro M, Kim I, Huynh A, Fu P, Mann M, Popkin DL. The use of 3D-printed models to optimize patient education and alleviate perioperative anxiety in mohs micrographic surgery: a randomized controlled trial. J Am Acad Dermatol June 1, 2019. pii: S0190-9622(19)30889-8.

[21] Wake N, Rosenkrantz AB, Huang R, Park KU, Wysock JS, Taneja SS, Huang WC, Sodickson DK, Chandarana H. Patient-specific 3D printed and augmented reality kidney and prostate cancer models: impact on patient education. 3D Print Med. February 19, 2019;5(1):4.

The long and winding road from CT and MRI images to 3D models

2

Vassilios Tsioukas, PhD [1], Ion-Anastasios Karolos, PhD [4],
Georgios Tsoulfas, MD, PhD [2], Jasjit S. Suri, PhD, MBA, FAIMBE, FAIUM [3],
Christos Pikridas, PhD [5]

[1]*Electrical Engineer, Professor, School of Rural and Surveying Engineering, Aristotle University of Thessaloniki, Thessaloniki, Greece;* [2]*Associate Professor, Department of Surgery, Aristotle University of Thessaloniki, Thessaloniki, Greece;* [3]*Global Biomedical Technologies, Inc., California, United States;* [4]*Rural and Surveying Engineer, School of Rural and Surveying Engineering, Aristotle University of Thessaloniki, Thessaloniki, Greece;* [5]*Professor, Rural and Surveying Engineer, School of Rural and Surveying Engineering, Department of Geodesy and Surveying, Aristotle University of Thessaloniki, Thessaloniki, Greece*

Basic processing

Today, the extraction of 3D models of internal human body organs from a high-resolution series of CT scan images can be accomplished with the use of appropriate software that often accompanies the instrument of the CT scanner. Appropriate software connected directly to the CT scanner processes images stored in a specific file format created for proper storage, transport, and visualization of medical imaging data well known as DICOM (Digital Imaging and Communications in Medicine).

DICOM is the standard for the communication and management of medical imaging information and related data. DICOM is most commonly used for storing and transmitting medical images, enabling the integration of medical imaging devices such as scanners, servers, workstations, printers, network hardware, and picture archiving and communication systems (PACS) from multiple manufacturers. It has been widely adopted by hospitals and is making inroads into smaller applications like dentists' and doctors' offices [1].

Traditionally the main steps of medical image processing are:

- Enhancement
- Segmentation
- Quantification
- Registration
- Visualization

3D Printing: Applications in Medicine and Surgery. https://doi.org/10.1016/B978-0-323-66164-5.00002-7

The current document purposes are beyond the description of the above-mentioned processes to analyze and edit DICOM images. More information on the above-mentioned image processing steps can be retrieved from relevant literature [2].

To produce a printed 3D model from tomography images, the usual processing steps are:

1. Enhancement
2. Segmentation
3. Extraction model (usually semiautomatic techniques)
4. Noise removal and smoothing
5. Slicing
6. 3D printing

Although the processing of a series of CT scan images is, at least in the initial stages, common to the processing of individual images (e.g., enhancement, segmentation), there are two parameters that cannot be ignored:

- Direct georeferencing (registration) of each pixel of displayed pixel positions. The technology of CT scans is able to directly define a local coordinate system in each image by defining the step between slice thickness and pixel dimensioning (x and y pixel spacing information)
- Each image is connected and has continuity with the next and the previous one and the imaging of the sections can produce any other projection (axial, collateral, lateral)

The first stage of the processing involves the enhancement (usually in gray values) of the image that can define the boundaries between the different tissues depicted in each separate DICOM image. This technique involves transformations of the original image through filters (low-high and bandpass filters, edge detection-enhancement filters, etc.)

In the second step, some transformations are applied, and the goal is to group together the pixels in each DICOM image so that each group gathers pixels depicting the same material (bones, muscles, fat, vessels). The process is often called classification, and simple filters or advanced statistical analysis techniques (k-means clustering, supervised classification, support vector machine classification, etc.) can be used. It is the most important and difficult step of processing since the success of the grouping of pixel in separate volumes belonging to different organs will define the success of the 3D model production.

The third processing step involves connecting all pixels of the same group from successive DICOM images in a file describing the 3D information of an object.

Again, it is necessary to apply methods of enhancing and noise removal (normalization, generalization, etc.) in the final 3D model object. This is implemented within the task of the fourth processing step.

The final model can be visualized in appropriate software and sent to a 3D printer for the creation of the tangible object.

In the fifth stage, the 3D model file will again be processed (converted from 3D) into sequential 2D layers (representing a horizontal section-layer of the object). This process is called slicing and breaks the 3D model into 2D slices using appropriate software (Slicer).

In the sixth and final stage, printing with the appropriate printer and the appropriate material (described below) will take place. The printing may need a small number of days to finish.

As it was described earlier the most important stage of processing to extract the 3D model of a specific part of the human body and specially to perform its isolation from adjacent tissues is an easy process and quite automated in some cases, whereas in other cases the process requires manual operations that often require a one by one image processing approach for the complete set of CT scan images.

For example, if it is necessary to create a model of a bone or a surface area that are very well separated from the soft tissues (skin, muscle, fat, and so on), the process is simple and easy. All that is required is the determination (usually manual or sometimes with a predetermined value) of the threshold density above which a tissue is designated as bone, or blood vessel. Below this threshold value, the pixel (or better voxel—volume element) is indifferent and should not be included in the geometry of the model.

Any software that connects and drives a CT scanner is accompanied by appropriate software that can be produced by applying all of the above techniques for noise removal, enhancement, segmentation, and visualization of the results for extracting internal human body organ, but within the basic configuration only threshold and simple image enhancement procedures are installed. Frequently, there is no capability to extract from specialized CT scan software the complete 3D models of complicate internal human body organs (for example, liver, pancreas).

The following paragraphs are dedicated to the two best practice approaches to extract from DICOM images 3D models of either bones or internal human body organs (in our case the liver). Our study is concentrated to open-source generic software applications since our study is addressed to people who may not have access to commercial software applications that are probably attached to CT scanners, performing special algorithms on the produced images.

Best practices
3D slicer

3D Slicer is an open-source software platform for medical image informatics, image processing, and three-dimensional visualization. Built over two decades through support from the National Institutes of Health and a worldwide developer community, Slicer brings free, powerful cross-platform processing tools to physicians, researchers, and the general public [3].

The software has very good documentation of both basic and specialized functions [4] and specifically to produce models for 3D printing [5].

A typical flowchart of image processing for creating semiautomatic processes for producing a model for printing is the following:

- Import images in DICOM format
- Load images
- Definition of clipping area (defined as crop volume process)
- Perform segmentation (add segments)
  - Set the isolation threshold
  - Removing noise in speckle and islands
  - Cut off unwanted structures
- Visualization of results
- Save to a suitable 3D print file

The software has a lot of features and ways to visualize both different projections of a CT or MRI scan and is also available for researchers to contribute providing their own solution.

To produce a spine part model the processing did not take more than 10 minutes interaction with the system (Figs. 2.1 and 2.2). Of course, it depends on the complexity of the model to be generated how much time it will take to provide the final model.

MiTK

The Medical Imaging Interaction Toolkit (MiTK) is a free open-source software system for development of interactive medical image processing software. MiTK combines the Insight Toolkit (ITK) and the Visualization Toolkit (VTK) with an application framework. As a toolkit, MiTK offers those features that are relevant

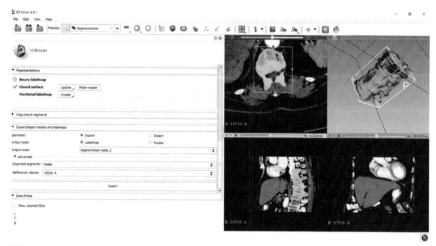

FIGURE 2.1

Workspace in 3D Slicer during the production of 3D bone model and specific part of the spine from CT.

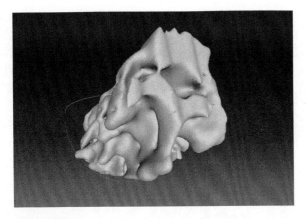

FIGURE 2.2

Derived 3D model from 3D Slicer ready to print.

for the development of interactive medical imaging software covered neither by ITK nor by VTK; see the Toolkit Features for details [6].

In fact, this is a DICOM image data processing library that can be embedded in software designed and implemented using different programming languages (C/C++, python) and on different operating systems (Windows, MacOs, Linux). In addition to the ability to integrate features from the toolkit, there exists a distribution offering an integrated processing environment with the brand name MiTK Work-Bench. A very recent development of this Toolkit platform and the WorkBench is the integration of Artificial Intelligence (AI) algorithms to export models of volumes from CT images and to produce the 3D models of internal human body organs. The problem of isolating the tissues of an internal human body organ lies in its vague geometry (shape, size) that an individual can have and in the proximity to other body parts that may have similar characteristics and therefore same density and gray scale value in DICOM images.

To perform the determination of an internal human body organ model, with the minimum interaction, the process is quite easy to follow (Fig. 2.3). The software just needs the collection of at least six points covering its most extend the boundaries of the human organ with other parts of the body. It is also feasible to follow proper corrections and revisit the solution with a better approach.

The software is also supported with the detailed documentation and tutorials [7].

Artificial intelligence features have been developed and built into NVIDIA graphics cards, and specific NVIDIA AGX and DGX Systems are not only capable of using predefined function algorithms to extract 3D and other information from DICOM images, but also to be "trained" (following a proper training procedure) to extract the appropriate and customized data from a CT scanned image series [8].

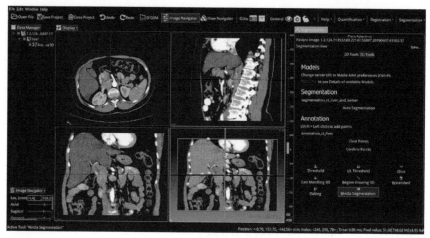

FIGURE 2.3

The extraction of the liver of a patient is a quite easy process. It needs just the collection of at least six points on the liver boundary with other organs to determine automatically its geometry.

Pilot case study

In July 2019, at the Aristotle University of Thessaloniki and more specifically at the 1st University Surgical Clinic, for the first time in Greece, a printed 3D model was used to aid a difficult surgery for the removal of a single tumor from a patient suffering from liver cancer. CT scanner examinations were used to evaluate and estimate the extent of the patient's illness at the General Hospital of Thessaloniki "Papageorgiou." The CT scans were performed in a very high spatial resolution (0.71 mm in XYZ dimension) and in three phases (portal, delayed, arterial) in order to extract the patient's liver model with the highest accuracy.

The CT scan images were then processed and the tumor and liver models were extracted using MiTK Workbench using the AI algorithms (CLARA) built into an NVIDIA graphics card. The connection of the MiTK Workbench software with the embedded library of functions of the graphics card was made via the Internet connection with a Linux server where the hardware was originally installed.

Liver parenchyma and tumor models were extracted into separate files (Fig. 2.4) and were printed for time-saving purposes in two different 3D printers but with the same characteristics in different colors and in 1:1 scale (Fig. 2.5A—D).

Liver parenchyma print time was approximately 2 days and for the tumor it was 4 h. The final assembled physical model (Fig. 2.5C and D) was used as to help the surgical process. It gave a clear picture of the tumor and helped the improved planning of the surgery by the physicians, as well as the increased understanding of the difficulty of the surgery by the patient and the family. The material used to print the models was colored (purple and green) PLA, while natural printing PVA was used to support printing (Fig. 2.6). The model of the printers used was the Ultimate S5

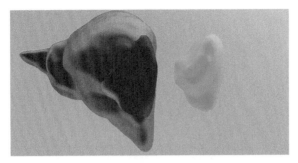

FIGURE 2.4

Liver parenchyma in purple and tumor in green.

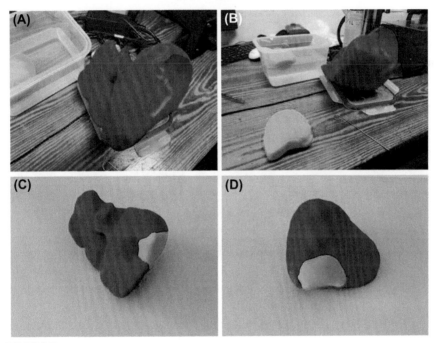

FIGURE 2.5

(A) Printer model of liver parenchyma. (B) Model of tumor and parenchyma. (C) Assembly of the two models (for bottom view). (D) Assembly of the two models (for top view).

which has been described as the Best Dual Extruder 3D Printer FDM of summer 2019.

The research and more specifically the tasks of the 3D modeling extraction, printing, surgery planning, and surgery assessment are part of the research program with the acronym "**Liver3D**" which is cofinanced by the European Union and Greek national funds and has a duration of 3 years (July 2018 until July 2021).

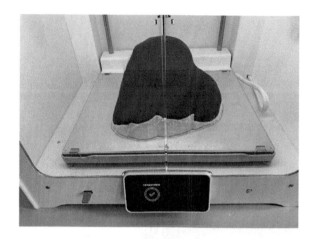

FIGURE 2.6

Natural PVA (white material) was used to support hanging parts of the liver parenchyma model (purple).

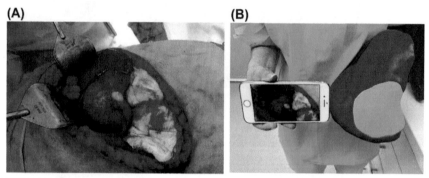

FIGURE 2.7

(A) and (B) Surgery images and comparison of printed model with the tumor picture.

After the surgery, the doctors evaluated the operation and the success of planning by numerical calculations (Fig. 2.7A and B). The part of the liver and tumor extracted from the liver was measured using 3D recording techniques (Fig. 2.8) and more specifically the combination of Structure by Occipital and iPad [9].

3D printers and materials

The most common types of devices that have so far been used for the wide production of prototype print models are described in the next paragraphs [10].

Extrusion material (fused deposition modeling)

The material extrusion technique is the most affordable at the cost of both the printing device and consumables. It is available in a variety of sizes of the printing table

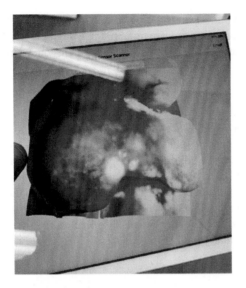

FIGURE 2.8

Capture model with Structure on Ipad.

(a typical size covers a cube of approximately $20 \times 20 \times 20$cm) and has been designed for special applications for printers that can even build fully functional buildings (mostly small single story houses). The material used is usually in the form of a plastic fiber which is heated at high temperature (e.g., 200°C), and it is directed through the extruder at the appropriate location for the creation, in successive levels, of a 3D form (Fig. 2.9). The most common materials that are used are

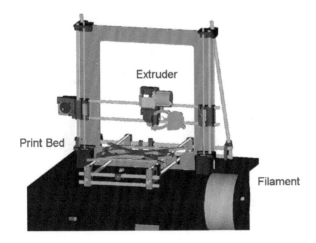

FIGURE 2.9

FDM Printer.

polylactic acid (PLA) or acrylonitrile butadiene styrene (ABS), while in some cases nylon, glass, ceramic, or other plastic material may be used which is initially heated and placed on the heated bed in fluid form and then, via a physical process (e.g., cooling) it solidifies.

Vat photopolymerization (SLA/DLP)

The technique of vat photopolymerization is also referred to as stereolithography (SLA) or as Digital Light Processing (DLP). The device is separated into three main parts: a high-intensity (ultraviolet) light source, a reservoir or tray of epoxy or acrylic resin that can be solidified after proper processing, and a control system that directs the light beam for selective illumination of the upper layer of the resin. The top resin layer is advanced successively perpendicular to the vertical axis and is exposed to the ultraviolet light source in the cross-sectional shape of the model to be manufactured. As the resin hardens under the effect of the light beam, the shape of the 3D model is gradually built (Fig. 2.10).

Power bed fusion

This category of 3D printing technologies uses SLS (selective laser sintering), direct metal laser sintering (DMLS), selective laser melting (SLM), or electron beam melting (EBM). All these technologies use a high-powered laser beam or electron beam to melt small particles (in powder form) of plastic, metal, ceramic, or glass inside the printing device in a special bucket. The powder is usually preheated to temperatures just below the melting point of the material. Thereafter, the power source is controlled by the printer, allowing it to selectively melt any successive layer of powder on the surface of the drum. After the first layer has melted, the powder bin is lowered and a new layer of material is placed at the top by a feeder; hence a

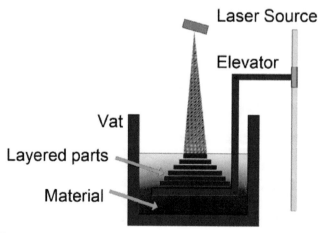

FIGURE 2.10

Vat Photopolymerization printer.

new layer is ready for melting. The bucket is always filled with material as the melting and welding process continues and there is no need to create support prints; therefore, it is much easier and faster to construct complicated shapes and in particular medical implants.

Material jetting

Material jetting is a different technology much associated with vat photopolymerization as it is based on hardening radiation, but it also follows the principles of conventional inkjet printing. While inkjet printers print ink on paper that dries and leaves the desired footprint, 3D inkjet printers instead of dropping paper ink, drop liquid layers that are exposed under light rays on a special UV tray. Layers are "built" one at a time to create a three-dimensional model. Fully processed models can just be printed and can be used directly without additional processing. In addition to the desirable materials that make up the model, the 3D printer appropriately uses a gel-type support material specifically designed to support overhangs of the model and other complex geometries that are easily removed by hand and water. Inkjet printing technology has many advantages for the rapid construction of prototypes, with superior quality, high geometric precision, and a very wide variety of materials and texture. Printers have unique technology that can use multiple materials in a single print. This means that it is possible to selectively combine different materials in a prototype print and even combine two different materials to create new composites with distinct but predictable properties. Many printers can use more materials and produce combinations of rigid or elastic and opaque to fully transparent characteristics, so that finished products can match the appearance, feel, and operation of even the most complex objects. In particular, for the reproduction of three-dimensional medical models, these printers supply a unique technique for the production, with the optimal quality, of 3D tissue models that can lead to a novel simulation technique well known as biomimetics.

Slicing and printing

The last stage for the generation of a 3D model is the process of slicing. This is also a very important stage of the process since it is connected to the final accuracy of the printed model and is related to the features of the specific 3D printer model used. We will describe only the concept for the transition of the 3D solid object file model to 2D slices that are given as commands in a file for the printer. For more information about accuracy and restrictions of the slicing process, the reader can refer to relevant literature [11,12]. The most commonly used slicers are:

- UltimakerCura
- PrusaSlicer
- Slic3r
- Simplify3D
- KISSlicer

Most of these are open source while commercial licenses also exist.

```
facet normal ninjnk
    outer loop
            vertex v1x v1y v1z
            vertex v2x v2y v2z
            vertex v3x v3y v3z
    endloop
    endfacet
```

FIGURE 2.11

3D object model geometry.

```
G81     X1.45     Y1.54     R 1     Z.25     F12
X2.5    Y3.5
X3.5
```

FIGURE 2.12

Commands in g-code format. These commands direct the head to follow the shortest path to arrive at the cartesian coordinates given as arguments to the commands.

An original object model is described with a large number of triangles whose coordinates are stored in a special format (Fig. 2.5). Everyone of the defined vertex (Fig. 2.11) is a triangle used to supply a part of the outer surface of an object. Usually, there is a connection (common edge) among two triangles, and under this condition the complete model of an object is defined by a closed shape.

However, the 3D printer, in order to be able to produce the model, should receive directions from a special driving file, which is constituted by a list of commands in g-code format (Fig. 2.12).

G-code is a language in which computer users instruct computerized machine tools to make something. The "way to move and act" is defined by g-code instructions provided to a machine controller (in our case a 3D printer) that tells the motors where to move, how fast to move, and what path to follow. The g-code language originally was used to drive cutting machines. Two most common situations are that, within a machine tool a cutting tool is moved according to these instructions through a toolpath cutting away material to leave only the finished workpiece and/or an unfinished workpiece is precisely positioned in any of up to nine axes around the three dimensions relative to a toolpath, and either or both can move relative to each other. The same concept also extends to noncutting tools such as forming or burnishing tools, photoplotting, additive methods such as 3D printing, and measuring instruments [13].

Therefore, commands included in an appropriate, for the 3D printer, g-code file give the instruction to move the head to specific X and Y positions by means of special motors. After the head is positioned at the correct coordinates, the material starts to flow and at the same time the head moves to create a horizontal section of the print model. When all material has been placed for a specific layer at a certain height from the base of the model to be produced, the print table moves downward to continue printing the next layer until finally the complete model is printed starting from the base and ending at the top.

Conclusions

Through the current study we came to the conclusion that it is already feasible to create realistic high accuracy printed models of human body parts that can be used for planning, training, and informative purposes.

The 3D model that was printed for the assistance of a very difficult surgery (resection of a hepatic cancer) has a threefold purpose:

1) To help doctors plan the surgery using a tangible and most important 3D copy of a human body organ. There is huge difference among the way that a physician (or any other person) is approaching to understand and provide a solution to problem that exists in 3D but sees it in 2D images (CT scan image). That is the traditional approach, where in all cases surgeons are studying CT scan images to navigate and perform an operation. Using printed models, the problem is provided in its real 3D extend, the physician is not making assumptions and the solution in many cases can be rehearsed prior to the solution.

2) The 3D printed models can be used for the training of young doctors and students of the medical schools. There is an undoubtable profit using the specific approach.

3) Finally, the patients are able to understand by touching and feeling the problem and embrace the solution to a surgical operation. Not only him or her but also the close family environment can benefit from 3D printed model observation and examination.

3D printing was not present before the 1990s and it is characterized as one of the fourth industrial revolution technologies. It has evolved very much since 2012, when the first low-cost commercial 3D devices came into the market (Fig. 2.13). It is just the beginning of a far promising technology, and more techniques that will be able to combine a big number of materials of different color, texture, and mechanical features will follow in the near future.

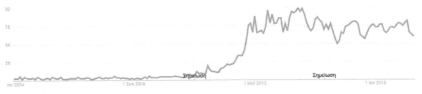

FIGURE 2.13

Google trends for 3D printing in United States.

Printing time is also in issue today. A typical volume of about $10 \times 10 \times 10$ cm may take 1 day to complete. Current research is directed to the production of more time-efficient devices [14].

We believe that 3D printed models using inorganic material are just a precursor of the 3D bioprinting technique that has already made huge steps to reproduce parts of the human body as fully functional internal organs. There have been successful attempts to create artificial skin or replacement bones or parts of them, but in the case of internal body organs like the liver the physiology of the organ and its functions pose significant challenges. However, the developmental pace is fast and the first results for the reproduction of a fully operational human body organ will appear earlier than we expect [15].

References

[1] URL1:https://en.wikipedia.org/wiki/DICOM.
[2] Bankman IN. Handbook of medical imaging. processing and analysis. Academic Press; 2000.
[3] URL2:https://www.slicer.org/.
[4] URL3:https://www.slicer.org/wiki/Documentation/4.10/Training.
[5] URL4:https://www.slicer.org/wiki/Documentation/4.10/Training#Segmentation_for_3D_printing.
[6] URL5: http://mitk.org/wiki/The_Medical_Imaging_Interaction_Toolkit_(MITK).
[7] URL6: http://mitk.org/wiki/Tutorials.
[8] URL7: https://www.nvidia.com/en-us/healthcare/.
[9] URL8: https://structure.io/.
[10] Rybicki F, Grand G. 3D printing in medicine. Springer Editions; 2015.
[11] URL9: https://all3dp.com/guides/.
[12] URL10: https://en.wikipedia.org/wiki/Slicer_(3D_printing).
[13] URL11: https://en.wikipedia.org/wiki/G-code.
[14] URL12: https://news.umich.edu/3d-printing-100-times-faster-with-light/.
[15] URL13: https://edition.cnn.com/2019/04/15/health/3d-printed-heart-study/index.html.

3D printing: shedding light into the surgical education

3

Georgios Lales[1], Elissavet Anestiadou[1], Vasiliki Bisbinas[1], Jasjit S. Suri, PhD, MBA, FAIMBE, FAIUM[2], Georgios Tsoulfas, MD, PhD[3]

[1]*Medical Department, Aristotle University of Thessaloniki, Thessaloniki, Greece;* [2]*Global Biomedical Technologies, Inc., California, United States;* [3]*Associate Professor, Department of Surgery, Aristotle University of Thessaloniki, Thessaloniki, Greece*

New three-dimensional (3D) printing machines have emerged, as additive manufacturing technology improves, leading to realistic models with accurate characteristics close to the real-life tissues. For this reason, 3D printing technology is gaining increasing attention from many institutions as an educational tool for a wide spectrum of surgical training. But this is just one of major applications of 3D printing manufacturing in medicine, as it is additionally used in preoperative planning on complicated cases, in helping patients understand the geometry of their problems [1], even for dealing with the empty spaces left after transplantation or amputation procedures [2].

This technology has been used in various surgical specialties such as cardiovascular surgery, neurosurgery, and ENT surgery to create high-fidelity models for surgical training. The extent of publications has led to the need for a more systematic classification and critical review of the data acquired regarding 3D printing technology. Addressing this request, the following chapter aims to provide an insight not only into the current status of these new techniques but also future perspectives throughout the different surgical specialties, as well as to discuss variables such as cost effectiveness.

Technical background

Before reporting applications of rapid prototyping for training purposes, it is prudent to lay out an overview of the consecutive manufacturing steps of these procedures. Data preparation, selection of printing materials and technology according to the final purpose are some of the key elements to take into account.

Steps of rapid prototyping process:

1. Collection of medical imaging data is a crucial step toward extracting reliable and accurate 3D models. High-quality imaging can guarantee time-saving and decent fidelity level of the final outcome [3] stemming from multidetector computed tomography, ultrasound imaging, magnetic resonance imaging,

angiography, cone beam computed tomography, X-rays, positron and single photon emission computed tomography. High contrast between structures of interest and adjacent areas is essential for better outcome [4]. All data collected are saved in DICOM format [3].

2. Afterward, the segmentation procedure follows. It includes the identification of the anatomical landmark of interest by selecting the corresponding voxels and, thus, marking a region of interest (ROI). Segmentation is conducted by software programs in automatic, semiautomatic, or manual way, and files containing the ROI can be turned into a 3D format through conversion to an STL file [4].

3. Additional model designs and modifications have to be done before final printing, which include optimizations such as surface smoothing. For example, "hollowing" technique is useful for fabrication of cardiac and vascular models, creating empty spaces through capturing and removing blood volume voxels from file during segmentation [4].

4. Undoubtedly, appropriateness and final utility of fabricated models rely mainly on accurate representation of anatomical structure or pathologic entities. Meeting this fundamental need, quality assurance and control of this multistep process have to be fulfilled [4].

5. Furthermore, postprocessing procedures will refine the 3D model as long as final control of anatomical accuracy is conducted, usually after evaluation by experienced professionals [4]. In this way, models can gain acceptance as training tools.

6. Final step is the printing process, in which many aspects have to be taken into consideration, such as optimal materials, multiple colors, overall cost, and time requirements [4].

In 1980s, Charles Hulk reported the first rapid prototyping technique, which was called stereolithography (SLA) [5]. Nowadays, 3D printing technologies have rapidly evolved and new laser techniques such as selective laser sintering are used. Nevertheless, even nowadays, SLA printing remains a valuable choice for medical use [5] (Figs. 3.1—3.4).

The following table contains basic characteristics of the most common 3D printing technologies implemented in recent years.

General surgery

Without any doubt, rapid prototyping has contributed in various teaching procedures of general surgery, particularly in minimally invasive processes. Steep learning curves in this field signify the need for 3D printing as an educational tool in this field.

Hepatobiliary surgery is a fertile ground for use of 3D printing as an alternative solution for visualization and hands-on training for the needs of medical students' education [6]. Nevertheless, concerns regarding complexity of liver parenchyma/venous/biliary anatomy and the need for anatomical landmarks have to be addressed.

RapidPrototypingtechniques	Fabricatingmethod	Advantages	Disadvantages	Layerthickness	Accuracy
PolyJet printers	Liquid photopolymers elaborated with UV curing	Wide range of colors, transparency, hardness	High cost of printer and materials Need for support material	At least 16 microns	+++
Stereolithographyprinters (SLA)	Resin elaborated with laser	Broad range of prices for printer and materials	One single material per structure Need for support material Moderate strength	At least 25 microns	+++
Selective laser sintering printers (SLS)	A basis of powder material elaborated with laser	Low material cost No need for support material Efficient strength	One single material per structure Extremely high printer cost	At least 60 microns	++
Fused deposition modeling printers (FDM)	Plastic filament elaborated by a heated nozzle	Low printer and material cost of Efficient strength	Highest layer thickness Low speed Only rigid models can be printed Moderate strength Need for support material	Thicker than 200 microns	++
Binderjetting printers	A basis of powder material elaborated with a binder	Multi-colored printing possible No need for support material Medium material cost	High cost of printers	100 microns	+

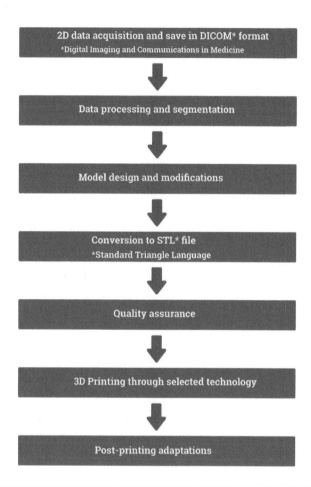

FIGURE 3.1

Step-by-step process of medical 3D printing.

Laparoscopic and robotically assisted hepatectomies in neoplasias and in living donor liver transplantations (LDLTs) are some of the training applications of 3D printing [7]. Two-dimensional (2D) imaging and intraoperative ultrasound are useful tools for hepatic surgical procedures, but there are limitations which can be effectively overcome by the use of 3D hepatic models in order to help surgeons acquire a better understanding of liver anatomy and develop hand-eye coordination [8].

An application of this state-of-the-art technology has been the recognition of hepatic segments according to Couinaud classification, which is a confusing classification system for many students and novice surgeons. A study fabricated three discrete liver models, particularly type 1: 3D-printed hepatic segments without parenchyma, type 2: hepatic segments with transparent parenchyma, type 3: hepatic segments with corresponding hepatic ducts. Each segment was colored in a different way,

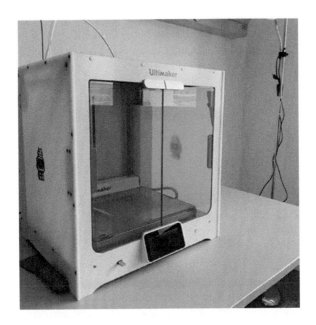

FIGURE 3.2

3D printing machine (exterior part).

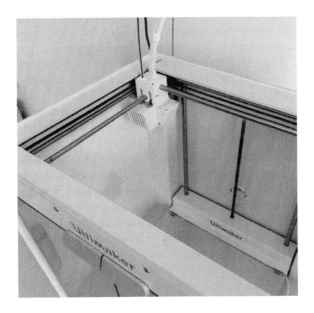

FIGURE 3.3

3D printing machine (upper part).

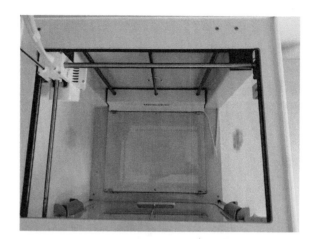

FIGURE 3.4

3D printing machine (interior part).

facilitating the visualization of liver segment architecture in three dimensions and also accurately replicating spatial relationships with crucial adjacent structures. Students' tests scores demonstrated the statistically significant impact of 3D hepatic segment models in teaching procedure, especially of the replica type 3, rending them useful to traditional anatomy teaching [9]. Deeper perception of liver anatomy and tumor characteristics through the 3D models could help eliminate some of the limitations of 2D radiographic methods [6]. Taking into consideration the significance of proper and in-depth understanding of hepatic vasculature for achieving successful surgical maneuvers and minimal complications intraoperatively, Watson et al. fabricated low-cost physical models of portal and hepatic veins of about $100 per model, abrogating the barrier of high cost. This study implied that these models can be introduced in weekly conferences, aiming to teach operative techniques to young residents and students, on the basis of following elective surgeries [10].

A great amount of 3D printed liver models reported in literature replicate liver and biliary tract structure with accuracy as well as common situations such as tumors, and thus, are used for stepwise surgical resection simulation [6]. Up to date, 3D solid models have been utilized for helping young surgeons and clinicians acquire proficiency in the anastomosis procedure during LDLT [11]. Javan et al. designed a novel solid 3D hepatic model of blood vessels, biliary tract, and pathological structures permitting the performance of hepatobiliary procedures. Via this, trainees were encouraged to practice procedures such as tumor embolization and biopsy, transjugular intrahepatic portosystemic shunt (TIPS) positioning, abscess drainage catheter placement, percutaneous biliary drainage and percutaneous cholecystostomy tube placement, acquiring confidence in dealing with hepatobiliary emergencies. Skills and simulation opportunities incorporated in training through

3D printed models so far also include laparoscopic gallbladder excision and hepato-blastoma management [12], while, Kagaki et al. were the first to fabricate a 3D printed hepatic model with replication of a perihilar cholangiocarcinoma, which allows simulation-training for the management of hepatobiliary malignancies [6].

Surgical resection is the most effective solution for hepatic metastasis from colo-rectal cancer. The advent of laparoscopy has initiated multiple pathways for hepa-tectomies resulting in a need for sophisticated and up-to-date hands-on training. Witowski et al. described the fabrication of a low-cost 3D printed hepatic model based on radiographic data of a patient, that was used as a guide for preoperative planning for a laparoscopic right hemihepatectomy for colorectal cancer metastases. Authors support that this model also has great potential as an adjunct of the educational process for medical students due to lifelike size and accurate spatial relationships [13].

Additive manufacturing has opened up new horizons in the simulation of biliary system interventions, since 3D printed models can represent specific disorders or anatomical variations such as common bile duct obstruction. Techniques requiring high level of expertise, such as EUS-guided biliary drainage (EUS-BD) of malignant obstructive jaundice due to gastrointestinal, pancreatic or peripapillary diseases after unsuccessful ERCP can also been taught on 3D printed models. Opportunities for training in basic maneuvers of this technique on real patients are sparse, hindering a continuous sequence of the learning process. Aiming to mitigate this challenge, Dhir et al. manufactured a 3D printed model of a dilated biliary tree by polycarbon-ate incorporated and replicas of blood vessels filled with aerated water in an animal liver tissue and examined the performance of clinicians experience in interventional EUS in four discrete maneuvers of EUS-BD, including needle puncture, guidewire manipulation, tract dilation, and stent adjustment. Trainees had the opportunity to practice on the most challenging steps of the procedure, maximizing educational profit. Materials were chosen so that the model would provide lifelike EUS and radiographic data. Each participant performed both the antegrade procedure and the choledochoduodenostomy. Consequently, participants were asked to evaluate the experience of practicing on the model for each one of the four steps and the quality of the radiographic data, but also the simulator's accuracy and feasibility to be adapted into the training curriculum. Results emphasize that this kind of novel seventeen bile duct replica would be a cornerstone in mastering ultrasound-guided interventions in biliary system, even without any further modification and also an inspiration for further models of EUS-guided interventional procedures [14].

Another interventional procedure with a key role in the management of hepato-pancreatobiliary diseases is choledochoscopy, which is considered a challenging process even for experienced surgeons. Previous endeavors included 3D printed models of the biliary tract and especially its spatial relationships with the hepatic pa-renchyma. Based on these attempts and on lack of previous 3D printed choledocho-scopy simulators, Li et al. used CT data from two patients with biliary system dilation to fabricate two biliary tree models using 3D printing technology for educational purposes. Simulators were evaluated by four experienced surgeons regarding accuracy and utility and then used by group A of junior residents for anatomy comprehension and choledochoscopy maneuvers practice, while group B had to study the same data through a virtual 3D image on computer. Outcomes have shown this choledochoscopy simulator to be a realistic and valuable tool for acquiring basic principles of the procedure, as it enhanced biliary anatomy and variation complexity and boosted manipulation dexterity and confidence of participants. In conclusion, similar innovations involving endoscopic procedures in the biliary system will be an important part of training curriculum of hepatobiliary surgery residents [15].

Apart from hepatobiliary surgery, the adoption of 3D printing technology for fabricating teaching and simulation models also constitutes an excellent option for other general surgery subspecialties. Transabdominal preperitoneal (TAPP) inguinal laparoscopic hernia repair consists nowadays the state-of-the-art strategy in management of bilateral or recurrent hernias; yet today it presents a steep learning curve and demands mastered surgical skills and techniques. Nishihara et al. noticed the physical inadequacy of current teaching and practicing status quo based on the apprenticeship model of training and tools such as cadaveric specimens and virtual reality platforms to provide sufficient proficiency to general surgery residents. To examine the impact of 3D printed models in training novice residents in fundamental but challenging procedures, Nishihara et al. developed an original TAPP laparoscopy inguinal hernia repair simulator composed of a 3D printed replica of human trunk and abdominal wall layers under pneumoperitoneum and handmade models of organs of the inguinal region, representing a realistic and reusable simulation station for repair of all types of inguinal hernias. Fifteen participants rehearsed in coordination with an endoscopist the basic steps of the repair procedure including management of trocars and hernia sac, mesh placement, and peritoneal flap creation and closure. Statistical analysis of answers to a standardized questionnaire revealed that incorporation of this simulator in resident training curriculum would be of great benefit, both for skill acquiring and maintenance.

An additional advantage regarding the use of similar simulators for laparoscopic procedures is the feeling of stress positions of surgeon's wrist, corresponding with accuracy to difficulties otherwise faced only in the operating room [8]. Apart from TAPP laparoscopic inguinal hernia repair, 3D printed models are gaining importance as a first contact tool of novice surgeons with principles of laparoscopic and robot-assisted surgery, rendering necessary the incorporation of minimally invasive techniques training in residency curriculum. For this purpose, UCI Trainer (UCiT) laparoscopic simulator, which is a laparoscopic simulator in connection with a PC or tablet device that collects training data on a platform, was designed and used by Parkhomenko et al. to assess basic laparoscopic surgical skills, such as peg transfer and knot tying. This type of simulation would be helpful for novice doctors who do not have the ability to perform and polish up their laparoscopic skills regularly, mainly due to lack of time or equipment [16].

Education on upper gastrointestinal system procedures is also a section of great interest, where 3D printed models are a sophisticated alternative option. Examples are gastroscopies and stomach biopsies, techniques mainly acquired through hands-on practice under the supervision of an expert. Lee et al. conceived and produced a silicone-based 3D printed stomach simulator with ten lesions for training in endoscopic biopsy. Parameters analyzed include total time required for taking tissue biopsies from all ten lesions, simulator accuracy to real anatomy and procedure circumstances and, last but not least, potential use of this model as part of stepwise training program. Trainees, including residents, first- and second-year fellows and faculty members, were called to perform endoscopic biopsy five times. Results highlight a decrease in time needed to complete the procedure, noted in all levels of experience and especially among residents, enhancement of basic skills needed, such as coordination with the assistant and equipment handling [17].

Another point of interest for further training opportunities of the upper gastrointestinal tract is thoracoscopic esophageal atresia (EA) and tracheoesophageal fistula (TEF) repair, which is considered an advanced endoscopic procedure with a steep learning curve. Barsness et al., after having fabricated a novel EA/TEF simulator repair with high cost and need for animal tissue, proceeded in producing a low-cost repair simulator of a C-type EA/TEF, which includes proximal EA with distal TEF, through 3D printing of the molds, filling them with silicone and placing them in a model of neonatal thorax. Trainees, both experienced and novice surgeons, claimed this simulator to be a flexible solution and a new promising tool in field of thoracoscopic EA/TEF repair training, especially for less experienced surgeons [18].

Furthermore, 3D printing could be highly useful in education of surgeons regarding colorectal and anal disorders. Arguably, anal fistulas can be a challenge in colorectal surgery, even for experienced surgeons, since they are accompanied by complex anatomy and route, close relation with sphincters, all of which may lead to severe complications and high rates of recurrence, even after state-of-the-art primary treatment. In the field of Coloproctology, Bangeas et al. was the first to endeavor to evaluate the impact of ten diverse 3D printed models of anal fistulas based on MRI images on anal fistula understanding by final year residents both pre- and postoperatively. Participants were divided into two groups, based on studying MRI images or the 3D printed replicas. After completing the fistula assessment test, residents who had studied fistula replicas achieved higher scores. Positive answers regarding other parameters, such as enjoyment, educational effectiveness and utility, originality and ethical issues were also more common among participants who studied 3D printed models. It is worth mentioning that the cost of each single model was approximately 3–5 Euros, enabling use of additive manufacturing technology for training clinicians in developing countries [19].

In the field of endocrine surgery, advances in radiographic imaging, mainly ultrasound and CT and ultrasound or CT-guided cytology examinations, have led to a significant increase in detection of patients who need to be treated. With regard to the field of thyroid pathology, fine-needle aspiration cytology (FNAC) contributes critically in the therapeutic decision and treatment and is necessary for nodules larger than 1.0 cm or with suspicious US findings and thyroid cysts. Herein, it is strongly advisable to assure accuracy, confidence, and constant skill maintenance of the technique, since it presents a high rate of complications due to close spatial relationships of the thyroid gland with the jugular veins, carotid arteries, and the trachea. Baba et al. used CT data to construct a cervix. The originality of this study lies in the combination of mold-based fabrication and 3D printing procedures, since the group constructed 3D printed models and filled them with polymers, mainly agar, so that organs of region developed after mold removal. This strategy assures that once templates have been fabricated, replicas can be easily produced, resulting in markedly lower cost and repeated practicing. Models produced were used by 45 medical students, residents, fellows, and thyroid experts for performing FNAC. The evaluation questionnaire revealed that all participants found the FNAC simulation model excellent for educational purposes and, also, a large number of medical students gained interest in thyroid diseases, resulting in a more profound learning procedure [20].

Neurosurgery

Additive manufacturing technology has broadened the horizons of neurosurgery education and training in a groundbreaking way. Especially in this specialty, it is highly important to have a deep perception of complex craniofacial and skull base anatomical structures, in order to be qualified and educated to manage challenging neurosurgical cases and procedures. A great variety of educational models, such as cadaveric specimens, live animals, simplified, augmented and immersive virtual reality systems, have come to light, in order to address the need of both open transcranial and minimally invasive operative skills [21,22]. Taking into consideration that opportunities for real-life practicing are limited, utilization of 3D printing on a large scale could assure improvement of standard neurosurgical and microsurgical techniques with a long learning curve, through activation of psychomotor skills [22]. What is more, future expectations of evaluation of an operator's accuracy and efficiency may be a valuable tool for recording technical progress and assuring the ability to execute a procedure on a live patient, preventing plenty of fatal complications [23]. Arguably, 3D printed neurosurgical models present advantages including low cost, robustness, portability, reusability, safety, reproducibility, realism and low cost-maintenance and storage needs comparatively to previous education methods [21].

3D printed replicas are emerging as a novel method for achieving state-of-the-art education and practical experience during residency in many fundamental steps, like head positioning, navigation, skin flap preparation, bone flap elevation, embolization, craniotomy, and lesion resection [24,25]. Ghizoni et al. report use of a low-cost prototype 3D printed polyamide craniosynostosis replica for educational, training, and simulation purposes, which enabled both teaching and understanding of regional anatomy and the various pathologic structures in three dimensions. It also constitutes a useful tool for training in bone maneuvers and refinement of surgical procedures such as fronto-orbital advancement, Pi procedure, and posterior distraction both for novice trainees and advanced surgeons, in a risk-free environment [26]. Moreover, Mashiko et al. constructed a hollow brain model with incorporated water manometer and a force sensor set on the spatula tool to train residents, through hands-on practicing, in mastering on pterional, lateral suboccipital, frontal interhemispheric approaches of brain retraction, an elementary step in creating a sufficient surgical field in every craniotomy [27]. Neuroendoscopy for admission to the ventricular system is the option of choice for managing obstructive hydrocephalus and performing biopsies and excisions of intraventricular lesions [28]. For management of hydrocephalus, Tai et al. presented the use of a rapid prototyping model for execution of skin-to-skin external ventricular drain in training seventeen novice surgeons, proving it to be an efficient, reproducible, and safe option in the training arsenal of neurosurgery [23]. Endoscopic third ventriculostomy (ETV) is a complex technique and a state-of-the-art surgical option for management of obstructive hydrocephalus, which is associated with life-threatening complications, such as forniceal injury, bleeding, thalamic and hypothalamic contusions [29]. Breimer et al. examined the utilization of an additive manufacturing silicone brain model as an ETV training station for neurosurgical trainees and pediatric and adult consultant neurosurgeons and reported its strong impact in advancing coordination and camera skills and thus promoting skills enhancement. Furthermore, this specific study included many extraosseous anatomic details, such as choroid plexi, mammillary bodies, infundibular recess, and the basilar artery and veins, as well as possible intraoperative complications such as hemorrhages, rendering this structure a realistic educational model [21]. Similarly, Waran et al. expanded the potential of an ETV training simulator, providing trainees the opportunity to perform at the same time an endoscopic biopsy of the pineal tumor, incorporated to the model [8], while the innovative combination of ETV simulating 3D models and special effect techniques permitted the visualization of a lifelike simulation station [24].

Unruptured intracranial aneurysms have a prevalence of about 3% of the general population, while multiple aneurysms are found in up to 20% of the patients [30]. In addition, incidence of ruptured intracranial aneurysms and following subarachnoid hemorrhage worldwide is about 9 per 100,000, with a mortality rate of approximately 60% [31,32]. Due to severity of cerebral aneurysms, there is a constantly emerging need for excellent acquisition of technical skills and related to cerebrovascular neurosurgery [33]. As a response to this increasing need, Liu et al. developed a 3D printed cerebral aneurysm model, incorporated with a skull and a brain model in a simulator, aiming to replicate with precision physiological characteristics, such as blood flow and pulsation pressure. This model was provided as an educational station for teaching the fluid dynamics of an aneurysm and also for training resident neurosurgeons in aneurysm clipping [34]. Furthermore, a 3D aneurysm model contributes in obtaining full perception and visualization of its three-dimensional structure, escaping from two-dimensional radiographic images [35]. Similarly, Mashiko et al. offered neurosurgery trainees and young specialists the opportunity to practice aneurysm clipping on a 3D printed model composed of the skull, dura mater, arachnoid membrane, a soft retractable brain replica, and an aneurysm with its parent blood vessel. Thus, the 3D printed aneurysm model served for training skills like dural incision, brain retraction, opening of the Sylvian fissure, and position of the clip in the neck of an aneurysm [36]. Fabrication of 3D printed aneurysm models used for educational purposes is also reported by Wurm et al. who utilized advances of 3D rotational angiography for this purpose [37]. Finally, Wang et al. produced a series of 3D printed models of middle cerebral artery aneurysms with various length, width, and neck measurements, so that novice neurosurgeons were challenged not only to perform mock slipping procedures accurately but also to decide the appropriate clip set preoperatively [32]. Apart from aneurysms, also rapid prototyping produced models which resemble cerebral blood vessel abnormalities. Dong et al. using data from computerized tomography angiography and 3D digital subtraction angiography, fabricated brain replicas with arteriovenous malformations that were used as a training tool for improving the comprehension of pathologic anatomy, the relationships of AVM to adjacent structures and the planning of surgical resection and endovascular embolization treatment by novice neurosurgeons [38], while they can be utilized by experienced clinicians as a training station for optimizing surgical dexterity [39].

Skull base and craniovertebral junction surgery and endoscopic endonasal, frontotemporal and retrosigmoid approaches for pituitary tumors, meningiomas, chordomas, Rathke's cleft cysts, craniopharyngiomas, and other neoplasms are another demanding field of minimally invasive neurosurgery due to steep learning curve, need for profound understanding of the regional anatomy and identification of anatomical landmarks through different approaches, and extremely high possibility for fatal complications [40,41]. Nowadays, training opportunities offered to young surgeons are extremely constrained, both due to ethical and safety issues inside the operating theater and lack of reliable and effective simulating models [28,42]. Shah et al. investigated the educational potential of 3D-printed model for recognizing skull base anatomical structures through a transsphenoidal approach, comparing scores of residents trained only by 2D pictures to those trained both with 2D images and the 3D-printed model [40]. Furthermore, Lin et al. through the use of 3D-printed personalized skull base models for two patients with a sellar tumor and one patient with an acoustic neuroma for preoperative planning, claim that similar models are a high-accuracy training tool, both for experienced surgeons, who can practice and adjust different surgical approaches, and for trainees, who can conquer step by step these challenging surgical procedures on pathologic models [43]. Similarly, Lin et al., through utilizing models of tuberculum sellae for residents' education, evaluated their contribution in shortening the learning curve of this meticulous procedure and their potential role in a trainees' training curriculum [44]. In addition, 3D-printed models are a valuable instrumental tool for individual skills needed in these approaches. Endonasal drilling is a crucial step of every endoscopic endonasal approach, due to the high risk of injury of adjacent structures. Tai et al. fabricated an endoscopic endonasal drilling simulator, which allowed residents to practice with the instrumentation used in the operating theater [45].

In the field of refinement of 3D-printed models as a substantial tool for neurosurgery teaching and research, many studies aim to increase the model accuracy, improving both anatomy visualization and the stepwise training. Favier et al. report polycarbonate (PC) as a realistic material for replication of human bone geometry and physical characteristics, in order to fabricate reliable skull base models for surgical skills training [42]. Nowadays, great pace of 3D printing innovations in neurosurgery education and training has also given birth to a novel multimodality 3D superposition (MMTS) technique, a fusion of multiple automated whole brain tractography (AWBT), and functional magnetic resonance imaging (fMRI) into a 3D-printed model. This advancement led to a better grasp of cerebral crucial connections and important functional centers, improved preoperative preparation, and increased skills self-confidence for residents and clinicians [44]. Last but not least, 3D-printed models have already established their groundbreaking role in neurosurgery training through utilization as equipment of experimental laboratories for microneurosurgery training, where trainees are able to perform surgical dissections on 3D replicas before progressing to cadaveric specimens [46].

Orthopedic and spine surgery

The advent of 3D printing technology has introduced a vast amount of innovations in the field of musculoskeletal and spinal surgical diseases. Together with cranial (12.72%) and maxillofacial surgery (24.12%), orthopedic and spinal surgery holds the lion's share of all publications related to surgical applications of 3D printing, with 48.16% and 7.46%, respectively [47]. First report of application of 3D printing in spine surgery came by D'Urso et al. in 1992 [5]. Applications of 3D printing in education and research in orthopedic field include the following major aspects:

1) take forward understanding of the complexity both of regional anatomy and pathological conditions, such as fractures, lesions or degenerative modifications
2) offer opportunities for residents' training, skill, and dexterity improvement
3) preoperative planning and surgical simulation

There are many reports and studies that underline the contribution of 3D printing in the theoretical and practical education of orthopedic surgeons. Anatomy teaching and research are main applications of 3D printing in the field of orthopedic and spine surgery. Accuracy and lower costs render 3D-printed anatomical models an emerging alternative to cadaveric specimens [48]. In addition, 3D-printed models through the visualization of complexity of pathological conditions, such as different types of structures, are a better educational tool than 2D radiographic images [48,49], while adjacent vital nerves and vessels render these models a valuable tool for precise maneuvers [5]. Moreover, Izzat et al. reported that surgeons claimed to grasp a more profound understanding of complex anatomy of patients with both degenerative elements and neoplasias, in comparison to other radiographic images [5]. Fabricating 3D-printed models with different calcium concentrations enables the accurate representation of the bone density spectrum [50]. What is more, McMenamin et al. report that 3D-printed models used for teaching purposes are able to give an accurate visualization of both structures of air and fluid negative spaces

[51], while Manganaro et al. highlight the emerging role of 3D-printed models on teaching hip anatomy and acetabular fracture classification [52].

3D printing has a great impact on essential skills needed for trainees and young residents. Through continuous practice it is possible to decrease the learning curve, complete a logbook of necessary operative skills using state-of-the-art simulation stations, and achieve better performance under stress-free conditions for the physician and risk-free conditions for the patient [50]. 3D-printed models can also play a profound role in evaluating a trainee's ability for decision-making and technique refining [53]. A characteristic example is the application of screw trajectory for intraosseous spine fixation, although the absence of soft tissues, discs, and ligaments lessens the biomechanical accuracy [48]. Javan et al. report the fabrication of a hybrid gypsum-based 3D-printed training model of the lumbosacral spine based on CT images, which will be a valuable tool in practicing techniques such as root pain management procedures, facet injections, and blood patching for managing intracranial hypotension, arguably challenging and demanding for trainees [54]. Another application of 3D-printed models in residents' education reported is the use of specific 3D-manufactured drill template to get trained in trough preparation as part of expansive open door laminoplasty [55]. Wan Kim et al. published the evaluation of use of 3D-printed acetabular models as an educational option for fracture pattern understanding and optimizing percutaneous screw fixation from 17 trainees' points of view, while using 3D-printed clavicle models. They reported the experience of trainees in selecting and positioning the optimal plate system [56]. Jin Park et al. also add the use of a real-size 3D-printed spine model for practicing free-hand pedicle screw instrumentation procedure in a precise way among trainees, reducing the risk of complication such as nerve and great vessel injuries and spinal construct failure in the operating theater [57].

Preoperative planning through surgical simulation has numerous advantages for residents and surgeons [56], enhancing surgical confidence through mock surgeries, thus permitting a better 3D understanding of the anatomy of the region [58], reducing surgical time and intraoperative complications, and optimizing surgical technique. Wan Kim et al. claim surgical simulation on 3D-printed model of musculoskeletal system to be of tremendous importance, especially for technically complex conditions and for novice surgeons [56]. Yang et al. comparing patients who underwent posterior corrective surgery for Lenke 1 adolescent idiopathic scoliosis patients with patients for whom a 3D-printed spine had been studied preoperatively, reported shorter operation time, less perioperative blood loss and transfusion volume, higher postoperative hemoglobin, and lower occurrence rate of operative complications [59]. Preoperative planning through 3D-printed models is feasible also for scoliosis fixation, including vertebral rotation, absent or dysmorphic pedicles and segmentation anomalies [5,59]; hemivertebra correction surgery; pediatric pelvic and spine surgery, ankylosing spondylitis; revision lumbar discectomy cases [53]; rheumatoid cervical spine [60]; patients with high-riding vertebral artery, irreduclanto-axial dislocation; three-plane proximal femoral osteotomies (TPFO) for deformity of the proximal femur as result of slipped capital femoral epiphysis

(SCFE) [58]; and spinal neoplasias [48], such as en bloc resections of primary cervical tumors, using 3D-printed spine models [50]. In all these situations, additive manufacturing, using data from CT and MRI, contributes to surgical precision and success [49].

ENT surgery

There is a wide spectrum of additive manufacture technology available to enhance surgical anatomy orientation and training in the field of otorhinolaryngology. 3D-printed simulators triggered a shift in the history of ENT surgical education, creating new paths in personalized interventional treatments.

Temporal bone dissection simulators dominate the literature compared to other applications [61,62]. Kyle et al. broadened their research on ENT educational models for surgical procedures through review of the literature until 2017, describing otologic, nasal, and laryngeal simulators. Models for practicing on congenital aural atresia, endoscopic ear procedures, auricular repairs, nasal and sinuses surgeries, and skull base interventions are some of the described subjects. But, as is mentioned, further peer validation is necessary for the above teaching tools. Training models regarding the laryngeal area mentioned in this study were anatomically normal and pathological models of the pediatric larynx. These simulators were assessed positively for high anatomic accuracy and low cost, but proved poor regarding tissue simulation [61]. More recently, another systematic review from Canzi et al. tried to summarize the literature regarding 3D-printed applications for educational purposes in ENT surgery, revealing that the majority of published studies focused on otologic models for surgical and preclinical education [62]. They collected 23 studies describing educational approaches in the field of otology compared to 7 and 5 studies in the fields of rhinology and head and neck, respectively. They also categorized the studies according to each area of interest, showing various simulators used for temporal bone dissection training and for endoscopic sinonasal and skull-based training.

Lip and palate cleft repair remains a demanding process with high surgical time requirements in order to avoid complications or morbidities. AlAli et al. [63] developed a teaching model of these deformities in order to assess its impact on helping medical students understand anatomic relationships. This study recruited 67 medical students from different institutions and showed that 3D-printed anatomical models of lip and palate clefts were superior to conventional 2D images from anatomy atlases. Although there are some limitations in the conversion of anatomic image data into printable material, the low cost of this model, calculated at $32, makes this technology more feasible than other options in being included into universities' curricula.

Regarding palatoplasties, a better understanding of the involved anatomy is the first step in the improvement of surgeons' knowledge. The next step is simulation of this surgical procedure in order to gain confidence resulting in better clinical outcomes. Cote et al. prototyped a silicone-based cleft palate model which was validated for its fidelity and utility as an educational tool [64]. Model characteristics such as anatomical and tissue compliance can be achieved without requiring excessive resources for manufacture, calculating the cost per model less than $10, allowing low-income health systems to include it in their training programs. Furthermore, they suggested high reproducibility of these models in various types of cleft, facilitating training on different surgical techniques. However, limitations were highlighted concerning lack of bleeding, muscular layers, and high time-production. This model was of higher value to novice surgeons rather than more experienced ones. Other limitations were the poor sample size of participants. Convenience of transportation is a key element of this novel model, promoting cooperation among many medical departments around the world, enhancing the clinical outcome even in developing countries [64].

A pioneering 3D-printed model of a patient's paralyzed vocal cords was presented by Hamdan et al. in an effort to visualize its complex anatomy, aiding the understanding of the challenging procedure of injection laryngoplasty. In this study, the essential value of this model in training less experienced residents in the technical aspects of the procedure was highlighted [65]. In some instances, such as advanced stages of laryngeal carcinomas, total laryngectomy is a considerable solution, leading, however, to loss of speaking ability. Tracheoesophageal prosthesis placement is one solution for this complication, although it remains a technically demanding surgical intervention. For this reason, Barber et al. developed an innovative simulator which would recreate the whole procedure of tracheoesophageal prosthesis placement [66]. The estimated cost for prototyping ranged from $15 to $50, allowing medical centers and educational institutions to introduce it into their programs. This study needs further validation not only because of its small number of participants but also due to its lack of follow-up data from patients who were treated by the simulator-trained doctors.

Esthetic, reconstructive, and craniomaxillofacial plastic surgery

Utilization of rapid prototyping technology in maxillofacial surgery was first reported in 1981. Nowadays, publication of the numerous applications of rapid prototyping in this surgical field place plastics and maxillofacial surgery second among other medical specialties [67]. In general terms, surgical procedure principles in plastic and maxillofacial surgery are oriented toward management of tissue defects, dysmorphisms, malrelationships, or a combination of them [68]. Furthermore, craniofacial structures, which are a vital part of daily plastic and maxillofacial practice, present with complexity and continuous need for comprehension [69], while meticulous techniques with a steep learning curve, manipulations of tissues with high accuracy and multistep surgical procedures demand the broad establishment of skills and surgery simulation. As a response to this need, 3D printing technology emerges as a powerful tool in the arsenal of knowledge and skills enhancement marathon. Computed tomography seems to be the best option for data extraction during 3D model production because different values in the Hounsfield scale correspond to different levels of tissue density [70].

A broad variety of pathological models based on patient-specific cases has been fabricated so far, in order to be utilized for virtual surgeries, giving clinicians the opportunity to practice on different surgical approaches and methods before moving in the operating theater. Apart from contributing to surgical planning, it enables surgeons to gain profound understanding of the anatomical complexity, spatial relationships, and manipulations of tissues that exist in the pathological entities replicated, to master operative techniques and to enhance surgical confidence. Models that have been fabricated so far for mock surgeries include cranial defect models of anterior skull base and frontal bone, craniosynostosis, facial dysmorphology models, mandibular deformities due to genetic syndromes or trauma [68]. Utilization of 3D-printed models for medical students and novice surgeons also has a more profound impact on their education, since it stimulates active participation in training without the compounding factors of limited sources and intraoperative stress. Last but not least, Schwam et al. underlines the value of 3D-printed models as instruments for educating nonexpert clinicians during medical missions worldwide [69].

Ueda et al., facing the need for realistic skin and soft tissue replicas for carrying out mock flap preparation and cheiloplasty surgeries, which are fundamental in microsurgery, fabricated a cleft lip and a face elastic model and with an outer layer made of polyurethane and an inner made of silicone. Some special characteristics of these models included replication of skin and subcutaneous tissue and ability for preincision marking, incision and suture making, and retention. Consequently, models have been used in training process, as six junior doctors had the opportunity to prepare flaps, one designed and performed bilobed flaps, while the second model came up to be a reliable tool for teaching the cheiloplasty procedure. The innovation of this group's flap model derives from the double layer, which enables undermining and suturing stably, in contrast to previous one-layer models. In addition, the visualization and performance of flap preparation in three dimensions surpass traditional training methods on papers or sponges, rending the practicing experience valuable and fruitful for junior residents. The low cost for these models is remarkable, which was $61 and $33, respectively [71]. Similarly, Calonge et al., using previous silicone of bilateral and unilateral cleft lip and palate models, fabricated mixture resin-based models for rehearsing simulation reconstruction surgeries by residents and for better understanding of pathological entities described in textbooks by medical students [72].

Rhinoplasty consists one of the most commonly performed surgical procedures and a chapter of significant importance in the field of esthetic and functional reconstructive plastic surgery. Despite the increasing need for mastery in rhinoplasty surgical process, opportunities for training without patient risk and at the same time preserving the educational character of the procedure are few. Zebaneh et al.

constructed a novel model for nasal hump rhinoplasty simulation with 3° of difficulty, aiming to promote training in fundamental principles of this procedure for residents, but also to familiarize medical students with the process [73]. In the field of rhinoplasty, Gray et al. designed 5 lifelike 3D-printed nasal replicas in order to assist 30 clinicians to provide insight into anatomical and biomechanical characteristics of nasal tip and also to visualize and get trained in reaction forces required during nasal tip plasty techniques [74].

In the region of maxillofacial and oral surgery education, 3D printing technology has achieved considerable progress. Werz et al. report use of fused deposition modeling (FDM) technology to fabricate patient lifelike surgical training models, taking advantage of characteristics such as low production cost, broad availability, accurate CT data extraction, and collaboration in production process. Specifically, maxillary models for external maxillary sinus lift and jawbone models for molars extraction training have been constructed, aiming to enhance comprehension and surgical skills of oral and maxillofacial surgery for young surgeons and dental students. In addition, materials used in models fabrication were also evaluated, finding polylactic acid to be a more advantageous choice rather than acrylonitrile butadiene styrene, because of its low toxicity and human bone-tissue fidelity during manipulations [75]. Another promising potential utilization of 3D printing is the enrichment of head and neck surgical oncology teaching process by importing 3D printing technology outcomes as an assistant tool to traditional methods and, in this way, improving the teaching quality and problem-solving capabilities, finally promoting rounded education and high-level technical proficiency [76].

Future perspectives of 3D-printed models in plastic and craniofacial surgery include the potential role of these tools as an objective evaluation tool for quantifying mastery of surgical skills during residents' learning processes [75].

Cardiovascular surgery

3D printing in the field of cardiothoracic surgery has been rapidly revolutionized in the last decade providing health professionals with improved means in visualizing common cardiac deformities and their relationships among neighboring organs and vessels. 3D models are nowadays used as supplementary tools of conventional imaging modalities [77,78]. This method expanded the understanding of congenital, structural, and valve heart diseases as well as the knowledge and experience in minimally invasive cardiac procedures such as transcatheter aortic valve repair via simulation approaches. Although it seems that the majority of published articles concern presurgical planning, there is a sufficient level of published material in relation to 3D-printed heart models for educational needs [78–80]. Future application of this technology would be to create digital data libraries to print rare cardiovascular malformations, providing the opportunity to multiple cardiothoracic departments to print and practice on such rare cases [77].

Congenital heart diseases (CHDs) are some of the most prevalent anatomic heart and/or great vessels deformities which appear in 9 per 1000 live births worldwide [81] and require surgical management at very early childhood to avoid mortality or morbidity [82]. Given the great complexity and variability of these malformations, congenital heart surgery can be quite demanding [82]. Recently, Lau et al. conducted a thorough systematic review including 6 studies concerning teaching processes with application of 3D-printed heart models (Costello et al. 2014, Costello et al. 2015, Olivieri et al. 2016, Jones and Seckeler 2017, Biglino et al. 2017, Loke et al. 2017) which showed the value of this technology in creating accurate cardiac models for training cardiac nurses, premedical and medical students, and pediatric residents. These models can also improve pediatric residents' learning satisfaction for CHDs and can be used for simulation-training for multidisciplinary intensive care teams [79]. Additionally, Lau et al. posed some concerns respecting the models' size and cost. Real-sized models are reported in only a few of the finally included studies and the cost ranged from 55 to 810 USD per model. A fabrication cost of 55 USD per model was mentioned by Biglino et al. but with unspecified 3D-printed model size. As the size is scaled down, the cost decreases, as does the quality and appropriateness of these models as educational tools.

Gaining knowledge regarding spatial anatomy is the first step to managing CHDs, while the next crucial step is to increase the surgeons' experience on the technical aspects of congenital heart surgical procedures. Simulation models play a vital role on practicing these procedures as Yoo et al. have reported [82]. They designed 3 hands-on training courses in which they used models of various CHDs such as tetralogy of Fallot, hypoplastic left heart syndrome for Norwood operation, double outlet right ventricle with subaortic ventricular septal defect. Fifty participants with various levels of experience on cardiovascular surgery, ranging from 1 to 30 years, assessed these models not only as helpful for augmenting their surgical skills, but also, found sufficient level of precision in each case. Course participants assessed the quality of the models as "acceptable,"' limitations for printing materials and disadvantages in structural elements such as cardiac valves were also reported. Overall, these simulators are discussed as valuable and applicable tools for practicing on congenital heart surgical techniques, thus giving the opportunity to less experienced surgeons to acquire confidence in these rare cases.

Myocardiopathies are common cardiac problems which under certain indications have to be managed interventionally by cardiothoracic surgeons or cardiologists. A very common example is hypertrophic cardiomyopathy (HTCM) particularly when it is complicated by obstructive phenomena as a result of the increase of cardiac muscle volume. Left ventricular outflow tract (LVOT) obstruction in patients with HTCM is a manageable condition which is handled by resecting part of the interventricular septum when there are certain indications. It is a challenging procedure but the variable anatomy of this region necessitates experienced surgeons or specialized institutions. Hermsen et al. have developed two patient-specific real-scaled 3D cardiac models from two patients with HTCM and LVOT mainly used for premyectomy planning and thus allowing surgeons to better understand anatomic relationships and practice before the procedure [78]. Although they designed this research primarily to examine its presurgical value, authors imply that this model could also offer positive educational outcomes for less experienced surgeons by flattening the learning curve. Therefore, after a couple of years they published a paper examining a curriculum program for practicing the septal-myectomy procedure which was based on lectures and 3D-printed cardiac models from the same material they had used for their previous research project. They reported promising results because the proposed platform gained the resident's acceptance in respect to the realistic models and the time and effort needed for practicing. They also noticed that the subjective characteristics of the resection procedure, such as the perception of depth, were additionally improved, with the participants matching experienced surgeons. Authors identified the cost as the dominant barrier for expanding their research to a higher numbers of participants [83].

Other cardiac diseases (e.g., valvular) remain common problems particularly in older patients. These surgical procedures need experienced surgeons. 3D printing offers a viable solution for practicing for both open surgeries and minimally invasive interventions. An aortic stenosis model has been prototyped by Shirakawa et al. using 3D printing technology [84]. They manufactured an aortic valve model using a rubberlike material and a hard engineering plastic material in order to simulate the soft normal tissue regions of the valve and the calcified deformities, respectively. This prototyped model was put into a porcine heart and was used by less experienced cardiovascular surgeons for training on valve resection and decalcification procedures. Apart from this, they used this simulator for practicing transcatheter aortic valve replacement (TAVR) procedures via endovascular balloon catheter. Authors reported a positive value of their model as an additional educational tool for decalcification training not only for the aortic valve stenosis, they also implied that this platform could be expanded on managing calcification diseases of the mitral annulus. The small sample of participants and their low-level of expertise (three novice cardiovascular trainees) were important limitations of this study. Especially, in respect to the TAVR simulation they described some concerns about the cases of more extended calcification damages, given that, the chosen patient presented low-level of calcification. However, this study remains a pilot due to the gap existing in the literature about the use of 3D printing technology as an educational tool.

Urology

In urology, 3D printing technology has been proven quite efficient as an educational tool. A lot of medical centers and institutions have developed novel approaches (models of the desirable part of urogenital system) in order to simulate major procedures which demand dexterity, such as the partial nephrectomy. These models were constructed from a variety of materials and thus have different features aiming to mimic the human kidney as realistically as possible.

Hakmin Lee et al. have constructed personalized 3D-printed kidney model from CT images aiming to assess the clinical usefulness and the educational outcome of these models. They concluded that both the urologist and medical students groups had a better understanding of correct renal tumor anatomy [85]. Other 3D-printed models which have a positive impact on helping trainees be more anatomically orientated regarding renal tumors are soft tissue models that were developed as part of the Maddox et al. project [86]. In this pilot study, researchers have succeeded in constructing patient-specific 3D-printed renal models with unique soft properties which mimic renal tissue features and used this model for educating urology residents on performing robot-assisted resections of tumors and renorrhaphies. The results seemed promising because practicing on these models helped the trainees to decrease blood loss during real-life surgery, shortening warm ischemia time, achieving negative margins in tumor resections and limiting complications. Tissue handling, cutting, and suturing accuracy assessed by experienced faculty members and residents with experience of robotic surgery conclude that model practice had comparative results to real-life surgery. This study also discusses limitations such as absence of small arterial and venous branches, lack of active exsanguination, and lack of perinephric fat which complicates recognition and protection of vasculature.

Most studies which have developed novel 3D-printed renal models used silicone materials both for its elasticity and its low cost [87]. For example, Monda et al. manufactured a silicone-based renal tumor model for training on robot-assisted laparoscopic partial nephrectomy [88]. This tumor model emerged based on the MRI of a patient and was judged satisfactory for training purposes. Participants of this study, students, residents of all stages, endourology fellows, and experienced urologists, deemed this model realistic and useful as an educational tool. Less experienced trainees have been proven to have had the most benefit in acquiring new technical skills, while it was judged of lower value for the improvement of existing skills. In addition, this pioneering training model was deemed more realistic for needle driving, cutting, and visual representation than for evaluation of kidney elasticity and tumor differentiation. For this reason, this model could be more efficient in the education of novice trainees regarding partial nephrectomy procedures. Silicone renal models could also be implemented on educational laparoscopic partial nephrectomy procedures, as they are useful for minimizing intraoperative ischemia time. Both reports stress the low production cost of these synthetic models compared to animal models, thus rendering it a more affordable educational tool [89].

A pioneering study with the contribution of additive manufacturing, fabricated a 3D kidney graft model and a replica of a pelvic cavity using CT images simulating the living donor renal transplantation procedure [90]. Kusaka et al. evaluate this system with respect to its value for preoperative simulation and intraoperative navigation and concluded that it could prove useful for better understanding of the relationship among surrounding anatomic regions, thus maximizing the intraoperative confidence of the surgeon and limiting potential complications.

Kidney stones are common in clinical practice and vary in size, with the largest being more challenging. Endourology is a field which offers dynamic solutions due to its minimally invasive nature. Leroux et al. in 2008 designed a novel model for training residents in percutaneous nephrolithotomies. This model was produced using rapid prototyping techniques and proved useful in teaching residents this procedure as well as for experienced urologists in planning more complicated cases [91]. Almost 10 years later, Ghazi et al. progressed to the construction of a 3D-printed model with the anatomic regions of the human pelvicalyceal system, kidney parenchyma, and neighboring regions aiming to simulate all the procedures of percutaneous nephrolithotomy with accuracy. Evaluations resulted in great scores regarding the realistic aspect of the procedure and recognition as a beneficial educational guidance for enhancing percutaneous renal access, nephroscopy, and lithotripsy skills. It also proved useful in evaluating these skills prior the actual intervention. Moreover, the superiority of this educational model is stressed over other technologies such as virtual reality simulators and animal models, not only due to its low cost but also because it has no ethical burdens [92].

There are many other applications of additive manufacturing technology in endourology education. The adult ureteroscopy and renoscopy simulator is a novel approach which simulates the procedure of catheterization of the upper urinary tract [93]. This platform was deemed anatomically accurate and simple to use by participants. It was also considered a quite useful educational tool by residents and suggested to be introduced into the residency curriculum. This model was deemed to have a low practice value for most experienced uteroscopists. Moreover, lack of bladder and urethra from this model and absence of physiological motion from patients' respiration are some disadvantages of this simulator, posing barriers to the extent of simulation.

Other surgical fields

Beneficial and innovative impact of 3D printing in surgical education is not confined among the margins of aforementioned regions, as the adoption of rapid prototyping technology by other fields broadens the dynamics of surgical education and training. In the field of obstetrics, fetal surgery through fetoscopic procedures permits the repair of congenital deformities without the hazards of hysterotomy. Notwithstanding, techniques required in fetoscopic surgery can be acquired only through constant training due to anatomical complexity and multistep processes. Miller et al., referring to the use of a patient-like 3D-printed model for fetoscopic repair of myelomeningocele (MMC), propose the potential future utilization of this surgical simulation for technical skill rehearsal of MMC repair [94].

Furthermore, in the field of anesthesiology and critical care medicine, there is a broad range of characteristic examples on incorporation of 3D printing technology in teaching and hands-on training. Flexible bronchoscopy is a procedure of crucial importance, and taking into consideration the high cost and the numerous resources needed for simulation of such multistep complex procedures, rapid prototyping is increasingly tailored for contemporary and efficient training. Parotto et al. worked on fabrication of a 3D-printed replica including the airway beginning from the trachea up to primary bronchi for providing the essential theoretical and technical basis to novice clinicians without previous experience on bronchoscopy, and especially by using and getting familiarized with real bronchoscopic tools. Parameters such as anatomy and technique understanding, accuracy, lack of local injury, time needed, and overall satisfaction level were recorded, underlining high degree of feasibility and performance and also an establishing low-cost bronchoscopy simulator [95]. Utility of 3D-printed tracheobronchial models is also apparent in newborn and infant bronchoscopy, where due to lack of time, limited cardiorespiratory endurance, complex anatomy and image restricted assistance encompass the risk of fatal complications. In order to meet the requirement for more intensive training on pediatric bronchoscopy, Hornung et al. constructed a 3D patient-based anatomic pediatric airway model suitable for repeated use, which offers extensive benefit both for normal anatomy and dexterity skill mastery and visualization of pathological entities [96]. Similarly, Fiorelli et al. report the potential use of a 3D-printed model already used for presurgical rehearsal on complex upper airway stenosis as a future high-promising educational tool [97].

Fueled by the emerging urge for continuous and efficient training of physicians in emergency cases, such as airway management maneuvers, in low-income countries with low doctor to patient ratio, a Cricothryoidotomy Skills Maintenance Program (CSMP) was established in St. Paul's Hospital Medical Millennium College in Ethiopia. The initiative included the use of a prototype laryngotracheal model produced by silicone, and its purpose was to supply unexperienced residents with skills on needle cricothyroidotomy and scalpel-bougie approach, in terms of low-resource environment and shortage of qualified manpower [98].

Another controversial point of residents' training curriculum nowadays is the numerous obstacles that hinder access to anatomy teaching and revising sources. A characteristic example is the difficulty with which ophthalmology residents obtain continuous contact with anatomy teaching methods, mainly cadaveric specimens, to maintain their perception of orbital anatomy in the time-lag between undergraduate studies and clinical practice. Reasons for this inconvenience mainly include practical factors (lack of time, no correspondence of possible study times, reduced dissections due to lack of volunteers, ethical and cost issues). Adams et al. have met this challenge by fabricating orbital models. More specifically, 3D cadaver-based orbital replicas of superior, lateral, and medial prosection approaches were constructed, containing significant anatomical landmarks marked with different colors and also realistic adjacent details, such as muscles, eyelids, lacrimal glands and apparatus, and cranial nerves. It is found that such anatomical models are a reliable, easily accessible, and accurate foundation in undergraduate, postgraduate, and resident anatomy teaching, broadening the limited potential of two-dimension imaging [99].

The aforementioned are at least some areas in which 3D printing technology seems to bring a new realm in the educational and training applications.

Conclusion

3D printing technology has proven its value as an additional educational method in several surgical disciplines. Better anatomy understanding of different pathologies and the enhancement of anatomical orientation among neighbor regions by novice surgeons, but also the repeatability of particular techniques which leads to gain knowledge, dexterity, and experience before the operating theater to the real patients, render this technology advantageous in terms of a better clinical outcome. As discussed above, more advantages are obtained by less experienced surgeons. For this reason, this technology seems as a beneficial option for educating the early stages residents, thus helping them feel comfortable and confident with several basic surgical skills and procedures. Cost and realism of the printed materials are deemed two of the main limitations in some cases; however, research on the field of 3D printing for medicine purposes seems to move rapidly bypassing these obstacles in the near future.

References

[1] Colaco M, Igel DA, Atala A. The potential of 3D printing in urological research and patient care. Nat Rev Urol 2018;15(4):213−21. https://doi.org/10.1038/nrurol.2018.6. Epub 2018 Feb 6.

[2] Sun DP, Lee LH, Tian YF, Zheng HX, Kuo JR, Wang CC. How to deal with the empty space after organ removal for transplantation: a single medical center experience. World Neurosurg 2018;115:e299−304. https://doi.org/10.1016/j.wneu.2018.04.038. Epub 2018 Apr 14.

[3] Rengier F, Mehndiratta A, Von Tengg-Kobligk H, et al. 3D printing based on imaging data: review of medical applications. Int J Comput Assist Radiol Surg 2010;5(4): 335−41. https://doi.org/10.1007/s11548-010-0476-x.

[4] Townsend K, Pietila T. 3D printing and modeling of congenital heart defects: a technical review. Birth Defects Res 2018;110(13):1091−7. https://doi.org/10.1002/bdr2.1342.

[5] Garg B, Mehta N. Current status of 3D printing in spine surgery. J Clin Orthop Trauma 2018;9(3):218−25. https://doi.org/10.1016/j.jcot.2018.08.006.

[6] Perica ER, Sun Z. A systematic review of three-dimensional printing in liver disease. J Digit Imaging 2018;31(5):692−701. https://doi.org/10.1007/s10278-018-0067-x.

[7] Witowski JS, Coles-Black J, Zuzak TZ, et al. 3D printing in liver surgery: a systematic review. Telemed e-Health. 2017;23(12). https://doi.org/10.1089/tmj.2017.0049. tmj.2017.0049.

[8] Nishihara Y, Isobe Y, Kitagawa Y. Validation of newly developed physical laparoscopy simulator in transabdominal preperitoneal (TAPP) inguinal hernia repair. Surg Endosc 2017;31. https://doi.org/10.1007/s00464-017-5614-x.

[9] Kong X, Nie L, Zhang H, et al. Do 3D printing models improve anatomical teaching about hepatic segments to medical students? A randomized controlled study. World J Surg 2016;40(8):1969−76. https://doi.org/10.1007/s00268-016-3541-y.

[10] Watson RA. A low-cost surgical application of additive fabrication. J Surg Educ 2014; 71(1):14−7. https://doi.org/10.1016/j.jsurg.2013.10.012.

[11] Baimakhanov Z, Soyama A, Takatsuki M, et al. Preoperative simulation with a 3-dimensional printed solid model for one-step reconstruction of multiple hepatic veins during living donor liver transplantation. Liver Transplant 2015. https://doi.org/10.1002/lt.24019.

[12] Javan R, Zeman MN. A prototype educational model for hepatobiliary interventions: unveiling the role of graphic designers in medical 3D printing. J Digit Imaging 2018; 31(1):133−43. https://doi.org/10.1007/s10278-017-0012-4.

[13] Witowski J, Pedziwiatr M, Major P, Budzyński A. Cost-effective, personalized, 3D-printed liver model for preoperative planning before laparoscopic liver hemihepatectomy for colorectal cancer metastases. Int J Comp Assis Radiol Surg 2017;12:1−8. https://doi.org/10.1007/s11548-017-1527-3.

[14] Dhir V, Itoi T, Fockens P, Perez-Miranda M, Khashab MA, Seo DW, Yang AM, Lawrence KY, Maydeo A. Novel ex vivo model for hands-on teaching of and training in EUS-guided biliary drainage: creation of "Mumbai EUS" stereolithography/3D printing bile duct prototype (with videos). Gastrointest Endosc 2015;81(2):440−6. https://doi.org/10.1016/j.gie.2014.09.011. Epub 2014 Dec 2.

[15] Li A, Tang R, Rong Z, Zeng J, Xiang C, Yu L, Zhao W, Dong J. The use of three-dimensional printing model in the training of choledochoscopy techniques. World J Surg 2018;42. https://doi.org/10.1007/s00268-018-4731-6.

[16] Parkhomenko E, Yoon R, Okhunov Z, Patel R, Dolan B, Kaler K, Schwartz M, Shah PH, Bierwiler H, Gamboa AJ, Miano R, Germani S, Fabbro Del D, Zordani A, Micali S, Kavoussi LR, Clayman RV, Landman J. Multi-institutional evaluation of producing and testing a novel 3d-printed laparoscopic trainer. Urology 2018. https://doi.org/10.1016/j.urology.2018.06.034.

[17] Lee S, Ahn JY, Han M, Lee GH, Na H, Jung KW, Lee J, Kim DH, Choi D, Song H, Jung H-Y. Efficacy of a three-dimensional-printed training simulator for endoscopic biopsy in the stomach. Gut Liver 2017;12. https://doi.org/10.5009/gnl17126.

[18] Barsness KA, Rooney D, Davis LM, O'Brien E. Evaluation of three sources of validity evidence for a laparoscopic duodenal atresia repair simulator. J Laparoendosc Adv Surg Tech 2014;25. https://doi.org/10.1089/lap.2014.0358. Part A.

[19] Bangeas P, Drevelegas K, Agorastou C, Tzounis L, Chorti A, Paramythiotis D, Michalopoulos A, Tsoulfas G, Papadopoulos NV, Exadaktylos A, Suri JS. Three-dimensional printing as an educational tool in colorectal surgery. Front Biosci 2018. https://doi.org/10.2741/13487.

[20] Baba M, Matsumoto K, Yamasaki N, Shindo H, Yano H, Matsumoto M, Otsubo R, John Lawn M, Matsuo N, Yamamoto I, Hidaka S, Nagayasu T. Development of a tailored thyroid gland phantom for fine-needle aspiration cytology by three-dimensional printing. J Surg Educ 2017;74. https://doi.org/10.1016/j.jsurg.2017.05.012.

[21] Breimer GE, Bodani V, Looi T, Drake JM. Design and evaluation of a new synthetic brain simulator for endoscopic third ventriculostomy. J Neurosurg Pediatr 2015. https://doi.org/10.3171/2014.9.PEDS1447.

[22] Suri A, Patra D, Meena R. Simulation in neurosurgery: past, present, and future. Neurol India 2016;64(3):387. https://doi.org/10.4103/0028-3886.181556.

[23] Tai BL, Rooney D, Stephenson F, et al. Development of a 3D-printed external ventricular drain placement simulator: technical note. J Neurosurg 2015;123(4):1070−6. https://doi.org/10.3171/2014.12.JNS141867.

[24] Weinstock P, Rehder R, Prabhu SP, Forbes PW, Roussin CJ, Cohen AR. Creation of a novel simulator for minimally invasive neurosurgery: fusion of 3D printing and special

effects. J Neurosurg Pediatr 2017;20(1):1—9. https://doi.org/10.3171/2017.1.PEDS16568.

[25] Kumar BS, Salem H. 3D printing in medical education a review of the current technology for future trends. December 2017.

[26] Ghizoni E, de Souza JPSAS, Raposo-Amaral CE, et al. 3D-Printed craniosynostosis model: new simulation surgical tool. World Neurosurg 2018;109:356—61. https://doi.org/10.1016/j.wneu.2017.10.025.

[27] Mashiko T, Konno T, Kaneko N, Watanabe E. Training in brain retraction using a self-made three-dimensional model. World Neurosurg 2015;84(2):585—90. https://doi.org/10.1016/j.wneu.2015.03.058.

[28] Waran V, Narayanan V, Karuppiah R, et al. Neurosurgical endoscopic training via a realistic 3-dimensional model with pathology. Simul Healthc 2015;10(1):43—8. https://doi.org/10.1097/SIH.0000000000000060.

[29] Kulkarni AV, Riva-Cambrin J, Holubkov R, et al. Endoscopic third ventriculostomy in children: prospective, multicenter results from the hydrocephalus clinical research network. J Neurosurg Pediatr 2016. https://doi.org/10.3171/2016.4.PEDS163.

[30] Etminan N, Buchholz BA, Dreier R, et al. Cerebral aneurysms: formation, progression, and developmental chronology. Transl Stroke Res 2014. https://doi.org/10.1007/s12975-013-0294-x.

[31] Hammer A, Steiner A, Kerry G, et al. Treatment of ruptured intracranial aneurysms yesterday and now. PLoS One 2017. https://doi.org/10.1371/journal.pone.0172837.

[32] Wang L, Ye X, Hao Q, et al. Three-dimensional intracranial middle cerebral artery aneurysm models for aneurysm surgery and training. J Clin Neurosci 2018;50:77—82. https://doi.org/10.1016/j.jocn.2018.01.074.

[33] Khan I, Kelly P, Singer R. Prototyping of cerebral vasculature physical models. Surg Neurol Int 2014;5(1):11. https://doi.org/10.4103/2152-7806.125858.

[34] Liu Y, Gao Q, Du S, et al. Fabrication of cerebral aneurysm simulator with a desktop 3D printer. Sci Rep 2017;7(February):1—13. https://doi.org/10.1038/srep44301.

[35] Mashiko T, Otani K, Kawano R, et al. Development of three-dimensional hollow elastic model for cerebral aneurysm clipping simulation enabling rapid and low cost prototyping. World Neurosurg 2015;83(3):351—61. https://doi.org/10.1016/j.wneu.2013.10.032.

[36] Mashiko T, Kaneko N, Konno T, Otani K, Nagayama R, Watanabe E. Training in cerebral aneurysm clipping using self-made 3-dimensional models. J Surg Educ 2017;74(4):681—9. https://doi.org/10.1016/j.jsurg.2016.12.010.

[37] Wurm G, Tomancok B, Pogady P, Holl K, Trenkler J. Cerebrovascular stereolithographic biomodeling for aneurysm surgery. J Neurosurg 2004. https://doi.org/10.3171/jns.2004.100.1.0139.

[38] Dong M, Chen G, Qin K, et al. Development of three-dimensional brain arteriovenous malformation model for patient communication and young neurosurgeon education. Br J Neurosurg 2018;0(0):1—4. https://doi.org/10.1080/02688697.2018.1424320.

[39] Dong M, Chen G, Li J, et al. Three-dimensional brain arteriovenous malformation models for clinical use and resident training. Medicine 2018;97(3). https://doi.org/10.1097/MD.0000000000009516.

[40] Shah KJ, Peterson JC, Beahm DD, Camarata PJ, Chamoun RB. Three-dimensional printed model used to teach skull base anatomy through a transsphenoidal approach for neurosurgery residents. Oper Neurosurg 2016;12(4):326—9. https://doi.org/10.1227/NEU.0000000000001127.

[41] Pacione D, Tanweer O, Berman P, Harter DH. The utility of a multimaterial 3D printed model for surgical planning of complex deformity of the skull base and craniovertebral junction. J Neurosurg 2016;125(5):1194—7. https://doi.org/10.3171/2015.12.JNS151936.

[42] Favier V, Zemiti N, Mora OC, et al. Geometric and mechanical evaluation of 3D-printing materials for skull base anatomical education and endoscopic surgery simulation — a first step to create reliable customized simulators. PLoS One 2017;12(12): e0189486. http://0-dx.doi.org.wam.leeds.ac.uk/10.1371/journal.pone.0189486.

[43] Lin J, Zhou Z, Guan J, et al. Using three-dimensional printing to create individualized cranial nerve models for skull base tumor surgery. World Neurosurg 2018;120: e142—52. https://doi.org/10.1016/j.wneu.2018.07.236.

[44] Konakondla S, Brimley CJ, Sublett JM, et al. Multimodality 3D superposition and automated whole brain tractography: comprehensive printing of the functional brain. Cureus 2017;9(9). https://doi.org/10.7759/cureus.1731.

[45] Tai BL, Wang AC, Joseph JR, et al. A physical simulator for endoscopic endonasal drilling techniques: technical note. J Neurosurg 2016;124(3):811—6. https://doi.org/10.3171/2015.3.JNS1552.

[46] Bernardo A. Establishment of next-generation neurosurgery research and training laboratory with integrated human performance monitoring. World Neurosurg 2017;106: 991—1000. https://doi.org/10.1016/j.wneu.2017.06.160.

[47] Tack P, Victor J, Gemmel P, Annemans L. 3D-printing techniques in a medical setting: a systematic literature review. Biomed Eng Online 2016;15(1):1—21. https://doi.org/10.1186/s12938-016-0236-4.

[48] Wu A-M, Lin J-L, Kwan KYH, Wang X-Y, Zhao J. 3D-printing techniques in spine surgery: the future prospects and current challenges. Expert Rev Med Devices 2018;15(6): 399—401. https://doi.org/10.1080/17434440.2018.1483234.

[49] Javaid M, Haleem A. Additive manufacturing applications in orthopaedics: a review. J Clin Orthop Trauma 2018;9(3):202—6. https://doi.org/10.1016/j.jcot.2018.04.008.

[50] Cho W, Job AV, Chen J, Baek JH. A review of current clinical applications of three-dimensional printing in spine surgery. Asian Spine J 2018;12(1):171—7. https://doi.org/10.4184/asj.2018.12.1.171.

[51] Mcmenamin PG, Quayle MR, Mchenry CR, Adams JW. The production of anatomical teaching resources using three-dimensional (3D) printing technology. Anat Sci Educ 2014. https://doi.org/10.1002/ase.1475.

[52] Manganaro MS, Morag Y, Weadock WJ, Yablon CM, Gaetke-Udager K, Stein EB. Creating three-dimensional printed models of acetabular fractures for use as educational tools. RadioGraphics 2017. https://doi.org/10.1148/rg.2017160129.

[53] Rybicki FJ, Grant GT. 3D printing in medicine a practical guide for medical professionals. 2017. https://doi.org/10.1023/B:RJAC.0000044110.16799.94.

[54] Javan R, Bansal M, Tangestanipoor A. A prototype hybrid gypsum-based 3-dimensional printed training model for computed tomography-guided spinal pain management. J Comput Assist Tomogr 2016;40(4):626—31. https://doi.org/10.1097/RCT.0000000000000415.

[55] Rong X, Wang B, Chen H, et al. Use of rapid prototyping drill template for the expansive open door laminoplasty: a cadaveric study. Clin Neurol Neurosurg 2016. https://doi.org/10.1016/j.clineuro.2016.08.013.

[56] Kim JW, Lee Y, Seo J, et al. Clinical experience with three-dimensional printing techniques in orthopedic trauma. J Orthop Sci 2018;23(2):383—8. https://doi.org/10.1016/j.jos.2017.12.010.

[57] Park HJ, Wang C, Choi KH, Kim HN. course_12_Chennai150323. 2018:1-8. doi: 10.1186/s13018-018-0788-z.

[58] Cherkasskiy L, Caffrey JP, Szewczyk AF, et al. Patient-specific 3D models aid planning for triplane proximal femoral osteotomy in slipped capital femoral epiphysis. J Child Orthop 2017;11(2):147–53. https://doi.org/10.1302/1863-2548-11-170277.

[59] Cai H, Liu Z, Wei F, Yu M, Xu N, Li Z. 3D printing in spine surgery. Adv Exp Med Biol 2018;1093:345–59. https://doi.org/10.1007/978-981-13-1396-7_27.

[60] Mizutani J, Matsubara T, Fukuoka M, et al. Application of full-scale three-dimensional models in patients with rheumatoid cervical spine. Eur Spine J 2008;17(5):644–9. https://doi.org/10.1007/s00586-008-0611-3.

[61] VanKoevering KK, Malloy KM. Emerging role of three-dimensional printing in simulation in otolaryngology. Otolaryngol Clin N Am 2017;50(5):947–58. https://doi.org/10.1016/j.otc.2017.05.006.

[62] Canzi P, Magnetto M, Marconi S, Morbini P, Mauramati S, Aprile F, Avato I, Auricchio F, Benazzo M. New frontiers and emerging applications of 3D printing in ENT surgery: a systematic review of the literature. Acta Otorhinolaryngol Ital 2018; 38(4):286–303. https://doi.org/10.14639/0392-100X-1984.

[63] AlAli AB, Griffin MF, Calonge WM, Butler PE. Evaluating the use of cleft lip and palate 3D-printed models as a teaching aid. J Surg Educ 2018;75(1):200–8. https://doi.org/10.1016/j.jsurg.2017.07.023.

[64] Cote V, Schwartz M, Arbouin Vargas JF, Canfarotta M, Kavanagh K, Hamdan U, Valdez T. 3-Dimensional printed haptic simulation model to teach incomplete cleft palate surgery in an international setting. Int J Pediatr Otorhinolaryngol 2018. https://doi.org/10.1016/j.ijporl.2018.08.016.

[65] Hamdan AL, Haddad G, Haydar A, Hamade R. The 3D printing of the paralyzed vocal fold: added value in injection laryngoplasty. J Voice 2018;32(4):499–501. https://doi.org/10.1016/j.jvoice.2017.07.011.

[66] Barber SR, Kozin ED, Naunheim MR, Sethi R, Remenschneider AK, Deschler DG. 3D-printed tracheoesophageal puncture and prosthesis placement simulator. 2017. https://doi.org/10.1016/j.amjoto.2017.08.0.

[67] Aldaadaa A, Owji N, Knowles J. Three-dimensional printing in maxillofacial surgery: hype versus reality. 2018. p. 1–5. https://doi.org/10.1177/2041731418770909.

[68] Pfaff MJ, Steinbacher DM. Plastic surgery applications using three-dimensional planning and computer-assisted design and manufacturing. Plast Reconstr Surg 2016; 137(3):603e–16e. https://doi.org/10.1097/01.prs.0000479970.22181.53.

[69] Schwam ZG, Chang MT, Barnes MA, Surgery A, Paskhover B. Applications of three-dimensional printing in facial plastic surgery. J Oral Maxillofac Surg 2015. https://doi.org/10.1016/j.joms.2015.10.016.

[70] Editors GTG. 3D printing in medicine.

[71] Ideas and innovations. 2017. p. 983–6. https://doi.org/10.1097/PRS.0000000000003764.

[72] Alali AB, Griffin M, Butler PE. Three-dimensional printing of models of cleft lip and palate:1-3. doi:10.1097/GOX.0000000000000642.

[73] Lederer R, Des M, Grosvenor A. Video ℘:952-954. doi:10.1097/PRS.0b013e3181b17bf5.

[74] Gray E, Maducdoc M, Manuel C, Wong BJF. Estimation of nasal tip support using computer-aided design and 3-dimensional printed models. JAMA Facial Plast Surg 2016;18(4):285–91. https://doi.org/10.1001/jamafacial.2016.0215.

[75] Werz SM, Zeichner SJ, Berg BI, Zeilhofer HF, Thieringer F. 3D Printed Surgical Simulation Models as educational tool by maxillofacial surgeons. Eur J Dent Educ 2018; 22(3):e500−5. https://doi.org/10.1111/eje.12332.

[76] Wei YP, Fan HX, Chen L, Zhang X, Yu JT. Treatments of second mesiobuccal canals in maxillary permanent molar: a report of 2 cases. Shang Hai Kou Qiang Yi Xue 2016; 25(6):766−8.

[77] Sarris GE, Polimenakos AC. Three-dimensional modeling in congenital and structural heart perioperative care and education: a path in evolution. Pediatr Cardiol 2017;38(5): 883−5. https://doi.org/10.1007/s00246-017-1614-9.

[78] Hermsen JL, Burke TM, Seslar SP, Owens DS, Ripley BA, Mokadam NA, Verrier ED. Scan, plan, print, practice, perform: development and use of a patient-specific 3D printed model in adult cardiac surgery. J Thorac Cardiovasc Surg 2016. https://doi.org/10.1016/j.jtcvs.2016.08.007.

[79] Lau I, Sun Z. Three-dimensional printing in congenital heart disease: a systematic review. J Med Radiat Sci 2018;65(3):226−36. https://doi.org/10.1002/jmrs.268.

[80] Moore RA, Riggs KW, Kourtidou S, Schneider K, Szugye N, Troja W, D'Souza G, Rattan M, Bryant 3rd R, Taylor MD, Morales DLS. Three-dimensional printing and virtual surgery for congenital heart procedural planning. Birth Defects Res 2018;110(13): 1082−90. https://doi.org/10.1002/bdr2.1370.

[81] Khairy P, Van Hare GF, Balaji S, Berul CI, Cecchin F, Cohen MI, Daniels CJ, Deal BJ, Dearani JA, de Groot N, Dubin AM, Harris L, Janousek J, Kanter RK, Karpawich PP, Perry JC, Seslar SP, Shah MJ, Silka MJ, Triedman JK, Walsh EP, Warnes CA. PACES/ HRS Expert Consensu Statement on the Recognition and Management of Arrhythmias in Adult Congenital Heart Disease. Heart Rhythm, https://doi.org/10.1016/j.hrthm. 2014.05.009.

[82] Yoo S-J, Spray T, Austin III EH, Yun T-J, van Arsdell GS. Hands-on surgical training of congenital heart surgery using 3D print models. J Thorac Cardiovasc Surg 2017. https://doi.org/10.1016/j.jtcvs.2016.12.054.

[83] Hermsen JL, Yang R, Burke TM, Dardas T, Jacobs LM, Verrier ED, Mokadam NA. Development of a 3-D printing-based cardiac surgical simulation curriculum to teach septal myectomy. J Thorac Cardiovasc Surg 2018;156(3):1139−48. https://doi.org/ 10.1016/j.jtcvs.2017.09.136. Epub 2017 Nov 6.

[84] Shirakawa T, Yoshitatsu M, Koyama Y, Mizoguchi H, Toda K, Sawa Y. 3D-printed aortic stenosis model with fragile and crushable calcifications for off-the-job training and surgical simulation. Multimed Man Cardiothorac Surg 2018:2018. https://doi.org/ 10.1510/mmcts.2018.018.

[85] Lee H, Nguyen NH, Hwang SI, Lee HJ, Hong SK, Byun SS. Personalized 3D kidney model produced by rapid prototyping method and its usefulness in clinical applications. Int Braz J Urol 2018;44(5):952−7. https://doi.org/10.1590/S1677-5538.IBJU.2018.0162.

[86] Maddox MM, Feibus A, Liu J, Wang J, Thomas R, Silberstein JL. 3D-printed soft-tissue physical models of renal malignancies for individualized surgical simulation: a feasibility study. J Robot Surg 2018;12(1):27−33. https://doi.org/10.1007/s11701-017-0680-6. Epub 2017 Jan 20.

[87] Smektala T, Goląb A, Królikowski M, Slojewski M. Low cost silicone renal replicas for surgical training − technical note. Arch Esp Urol 2016;69(7):434−6.

[88] Monda SM, Weese JR, Anderson BG, Vetter JM, Venkatesh R, Du K, Andriole GL, Figenshau RS. Development and validity of a silicone renal tumor model for robotic

partial nephrectomy training. Urology 2018;114:114−20. https://doi.org/10.1016/j.urology.2018.01.030. Epub 2018 Feb 5.

[89] Golab A, Smektala T, Kaczmarek K, Stamirowski R, Hrab M, Slojewski M. Laparoscopic partial nephrectomy supported by training involving personalized silicone replica poured in three-dimensional printed casting mold. J Laparoendosc Adv Surg Tech A 2017;27(4):420−2. https://doi.org/10.1089/lap.2016.0596. Epub 2017 Jan 6.

[90] Kusaka M, Sugimoto M, Fukami N, Sasaki H, Takenaka M, Anraku T, Ito T, Kenmochi T, Shiroki R, Hoshinaga K. Initial experience with a tailor-made simulation and navigation program using a 3-D printer model of kidney transplantation surgery. Transplant Proc 2015;47(3):596−9. https://doi.org/10.1016/j.transproceed.2014.12.045.

[91] Bruyère F, Leroux C, Brunereau L, Lermusiaux P. Rapid prototyping model for percutaneous nephrolithotomy training. J Endourol 2008;22(1):91−6. https://doi.org/10.1089/end.2007.0025.

[92] Ghazi A, Campbell T, Melnyk R, Feng C, Andrusco A, Stone J, Erturk E. Validation of a full-immersion simulation platform for percutaneous nephrolithotomy using three-dimensional printing technology. J Endourol 2017;31(12):1314−20. https://doi.org/10.1089/end.2017.0366.

[93] White MA, Dehaan AP, Stephens DD, Maes AA, Maatman TJ. Validation of a high fidelity adult ureteroscopy and renoscopy simulator. J Urol 2010;183(2):673−7. https://doi.org/10.1016/j.juro.2009.10.01.

[94] Miller JL, Ahn ES, Garcia JR, Miller GT, Satin AJ, Baschat AA. Ultrasound-based three-dimensional printed medical model for multispecialty team surgical rehearsal prior to fetoscopic myelomeningocele repair. Ultrasound Obstet Gynecol 2018;51(6):836−7. https://doi.org/10.1002/uog.18891.

[95] Parotto M, Jiansen JQ, AboTaiban A, et al. Evaluation of a low-cost, 3D-printed model for bronchoscopy training. AnestezjolIntens Ter 2017;49(3):189−97. https://doi.org/10.5603/AIT.a2017.0035.

[96] Hornung A, Kumpf M, Baden W, Tsiflikas I, Hofbeck M, Sieverding L. Realistic 3d-printed tracheobronchial tree model from a 1-year-old girl for pediatric bronchoscopy training. Respiration 2017;93(4):293−5. https://doi.org/10.1159/000459631.

[97] Fiorelli A, et al. Three-dimensional (3D) printed model to plan the endoscopic treatment of upper airway stenosis. J Bronchology Interv Pulmonol 2018 Oct;25(4):349−54. www.pubfacts.com/detail/30179921/Three-dimensional-3D-Printed-Model-to-Plan-the-Endoscopic-Treatment-of-Upper-Airway-Stenosis. https://doi.org/10.1097/LBR.0000000000000504.

[98] Gauger VT, Rooney D, Kovatch KJ, et al. A multidisciplinary international collaborative implementing low cost, high fidelity 3D printed airway models to enhance Ethiopian anesthesia resident emergency cricothyroidotomy skills. Int J Pediatr Otorhinolaryngol 2018;114(September):124−8. https://doi.org/10.1016/j.ijporl.2018.08.040.

[99] Adams JW, Paxton L, Dawes K, Burlak K, Quayle M, McMenamin PG. 3D printed reproductions of orbital dissections: a novel mode of visualising anatomy for trainees in ophthalmology or optometry. Br J Ophthalmol 2015;99(9):1162−7. https://doi.org/10.1136/bjophthalmol-2014-306189.

3D printing and bioprinting: ethical and legal issues

4

Takis Vidalis, PhD

Senior Scientist, Legal Advisor, Hellenic National Bioethics Commission, Attica, Greece

Introduction

The development of 3D printing applications represents a major advance in modern Biomedicine. This technology includes both the production of medical devices (organ models, instruments, implants, etc.)[1] and the replication of biological material (cell lines), that is, the creation of human tissue or organs via nonreproductive processing of original biological material (bioprinting).[2] The ethical aspects of these applications remain still largely unexplored.

There is no question that 3D printing, in general, may serve enormously persisting needs in contemporary healthcare systems, since it is expected to facilitate supply with necessary devices and material, making the whole process of production less costly in time and money.[3] Therefore, in terms of its objective, the new technology has an indubitable ethical value.

The future of bioprinting, especially, could drive to a real breakthrough in regenerative medicine and transplantations. Indeed, if we ensure that the production of biological material by this method guarantees, on the one hand, safety and, on the other, functional suitability of the replicated tissues, and even organs, we will be in place to effectively solve the problem of extremely limited biological resources for clinical use that we currently face (from hemopoietic stem cells, to bone marrow, tissue, and organs for transplantations, or even reproductive material).[4] This would be a new era for Biomedicine, as bioprinting could make possible the creation of a potential pool of replicated biological material with the advantage of histocompatibility for every individual. Ethically speaking, that perspective would serve by definition the fundamental right to health and, more generally, the right to our corporal integrity.

Yet the ethical merit of the 3D printing aim is not excluded from the general principle pertaining to any novelty in Biomedicine and, in fact, to any application in advanced technologies. According to that principle, no objective, whatever ethical, justifies the compromise of other fundamental values which constitute the supremacy of human dignity, as expressed in every person. In other words, even if our purpose is to serve the common good, by developing research projects that may be useful for society as a whole, not any means to achieve that purpose is ethically acceptable; only means complying with all fundamental values meet the necessary condition for confirming the ethical soundness of the research objective. In the law of Biomedicine, this maxim is repeatedly mentioned in international instruments, where the interests and rights of any individual are considered as prevailing over the interests of research, serving society as a whole.[5]

Indeed, particularly in the context of 3D bioprinting research and development, several important ethical questions regarding respect and protection of fundamental values, usually related to concrete aspects of human rights, need to be addressed. In the following, I will focus mostly on bioprinting to explore these questions, starting from their basic ethical conceptualization (Ethical issues section). Furthermore, I will argue about their legal understanding, with reference to binding instruments of international and EU law (Regulation and law section).

Ethical issues

Safety

A major ethical issue occurring in any novel application of advanced technologies is that of safety.[6] To make sure that 3D bioprinting applications do not create risks for the individual health of patients (and possibly for public health and the environment as well), we need to determine acceptable standards of safety for the use of replicated biological material. This is not entirely a technical matter, in the sense that the term "acceptable" presupposes an evaluation of available technical data, which encompasses also a certain selection between risks; safety standards eventually mean prevention of major detectable risks, even if we are aware of the possible occurrence of risks considered as insignificant or other unforeseen risks. To make that distinction, by suggesting a safety threshold, this inevitably presupposes ethical judgments about the risk "quality," which cannot be deduced simply by measuring biomarkers or other relevant scientific data.

Indeed the achievement of "absolute" safety is never the case for any biomedical novelty, as unforeseen natural effects may always emerge. In conventional clinical trials, for instance, aiming for the development of new pharmaceuticals, strict safety standards need to be confirmed in every step, during the research, until the successful completion of the trial and the grant of licensing for marketing the new product. Still, this is a short-term evaluation of safety issues, directly related to the reaction of the volunteers' organism during the trial phases. This does not cover potential risks that may occur in the long term, after the product's disposal in the market and its normal administration to patients, according to the approved prescription guidance. For addressing that problem, a standard procedure of pharmacovigilance for detecting such risks usually ensures a higher degree of safety.[7] This example is characteristic of the inevitable relative judgments on safety in biomedical applications, that is, the relative accuracy of risk assessment in relevance.

Following the above approach, in principle, safety management of bioprinted products should be addressed under the same ethical terms as for other known biomedical products (drugs, transplants, implants, etc.) meant for interventional medical acts. We know that, for such products, certainty of risks is crucial for determining standards of safety. The opposite approach, known as "precautionary principle," characterizes currently the application of novel technologies in the environment, particularly those involving genetic engineering, nanotechnology, etc.[8] These technologies are associated with high degree of risk uncertainty, due to the relatively limited level of our knowledge regarding fundamental biological data, such as genes' and genomes' interactions and phenotyping, details on the function of food chain, etc. To prevent unforeseen risks that might create serious and extensive harm to the environment, which could be irreversible, the "precautionary principle" requires measures to be taken even in conditions of risk uncertainty (including a complete ban of the concrete application), which is something more strict than an effort to positively detect such risks. The justification of that stricter approach of safety lies on the extent of possible environmental degradation, when a novel application is deliberated in the Nature. This is not the case of medical interventions in individual organisms, where the risks may occur to a rather limited extent, even if theoretically we cannot exclude wider implications affecting public health. Therefore, for guaranteeing safety in biomedical applications of all kinds, it is sufficient to detect risks in a positive sense, and take appropriate measures for addressing them, with no need to apply a "precautionary" approach.

Risks in 3D bioprinting are categorized in two main groups. First, it is necessary to ensure safety of the replicated biological material itself, if used in the form of transplants, that is, to avoid the possibility of contamination and emergence of pathogens that could compromise not only the individual health of the receiver of the transplants, but public health as well. Second, safety is involved in the functioning of the new transplants in the receivers' organism, that is, their suitability with the new biological environment. The first issue is already known from the field of xenotransplantations, where major problems related to pathogenic transplants (due to deep differences in the animal/human biology) risking generating serious infectious diseases obstruct such applications.[9] The second issue is already addressed in conventional tissue and organ transplantations. The difference with 3 D bioprinting is that there is no evidence that transplants produced are indeed functional, as they have never have been part of a donor's organism previously; their potential is to be tested for the first time in the receivers' organism, which might prove much more dangerous, even if the quality of the graft as such has been tested successfully.

Consent

The development and use of 3D printed and bioprinted products need to refer to the standard governing all medical acts, that is, the informed consent of patients. Informed consent ensures respect of the patient's autonomy, in other words it establishes personal control over the biological condition of our organism. The autonomy maxim represents a fundamental shift in understanding the patient/physician relationships, as opposed to the approach of medical paternalism, dominant for centuries in Western medicine, according to which the physician needs to hold full control and responsibility over the condition of health of a rather "passive" patient. Extensive changes occurred not only due to notorious historical deviations from the basic medical duty[10] but also due to the complexity in practicing medicine (given the increased degree of physicians' specialization, the rapid introduction of technology, and the availability of massive information difficult to be "digested" in everyday medical performance), led eventually to the recognition of an active role for patients (or, in general, for healthcare receivers) in their relationships with the attending physicians.

According to their new role, patients need to consent prior to undergoing any medical act proposed by the physician (regarding treatment, prevention, or diagnosis), with the necessary condition of appropriate information provided by the latter.[11] That information may include more options, which means that the patient needs to choose among these, orienting the physician's therapeutic plan. On the other hand, patients do not dictate that plan, as they do not have the option to ask for specific medical acts. Being the expert, the physician is always the one who has the responsibility to propose[12] and the nonexpert patient needs only to accept, choose or not, according to his/her preferences.

In that complex relationship, the physician may also disagree with the patient's stance, either for scientific or for conscious reasons, and abstain from the patient's care.[13] Such a disagreement usually emerges before starting the informed consent process, in cases where the patient requires a medical intervention unacceptable on scientific grounds or contrary to the physician's moral beliefs. On the other hand, after setting up the therapeutic relationship, the patient always has the option to refuse treatment, within the informed consent framework, if does not consent to the physician's proposals.[14]

Nevertheless, in emergency situations, where time is a crucial factor for the medical act's effectiveness, the informed consent process needs to be followed only in compliance with that condition. Thus, if there is no time to inform the patient or his/her proxies, to obtain genuine consent, the attending physician has a moral duty to proceed immediately to the necessary medical act, based upon his/her scientific knowledge and experience, with the sole purpose to perform effectively.[15] Still, even in cases of emergency, the physician needs to consider previous wishes of the patient (advance directives), if existing, as those are evidence of personal autonomy and deserve respect.[16]

Genuine consent and the role of patient education

A major difficulty that we need to address regarding consent is to confirm its genuine nature.[17] Genuine consent means that the interested person expresses free decision after having received appropriate information by the expert physician. Information should be complete and nonbiased to ensure freedom in decision making by the nonexpert patient. Even in conventional medical practice, that process presents problems, since no objective evidence exists to confirm physicians' good performance in information. Indeed, written documentation is not enough to check this; patients need specific information,[18] in oral form mostly, enabling them to pose questions and have concrete answers by their attending physician. Therefore, the quality of information depends on factors like the physician's selection of its important elements, according to his/her subjective assumptions, or the subjective level of knowledge and ability of each patient to understand and process these elements. Such factors are not measurable and are always suspect to facilitate manipulation of the patients' will, even nonintentional.[19]

Biased consent is often due to the information that nonexpert persons receive from other than the attending physician sources, mostly from the media. That is the case of novel biomedical applications, products of advanced technologies in biomedicine, including 3D printing or 3D bioprinting. The world of media represents the most eager promoter of impressive novelties, promising breakthroughs in Medicine, even if no reliable scientific evidence in relevance exists. The announcement of such promising applications, mostly by popular media, shapes the information that the general public absorbs, and forms a basic positive stance to most people, patients or not.[20] That portion of unconfirmed or even false original knowledge becomes problematic in patient—doctor relationships, when specific information on available treating options is required by the attending physician. A patient may object to conventional proposed options, if already convinced by a novel application, just because a popular anchorman or website has said so. This is problematic for the informed consent process, since the patient's prejudice in favor of the novelty obstructs communication with the attending physician. An extra effort by the latter is, thus, required to "clean" the patient's understanding from the false information upon which he/she relies, enabling appropriate transmission of reliable knowledge.[21]

That form of transmitting reliable knowledge by the attending physician, based upon a face-to-face approach, is essential, since a patient is more open to accept information by the expert he/she trusts mostly in the concrete therapeutic relationship. Yet regarding novel technological applications, such as 3D printing or bioprinting, there is no guarantee that the attending physician is always able to accomplish this role, particularly when educated patients have already strong beliefs about certain applications. Such strong beliefs are usually formed after personal elaboration of relevant information that patients have received from various sources (media, Internet, popular nonscientific articles, etc.). As the physician is not always familiar with that volume and details of information accessible by the general public, a need for developing strategies of patient education, with the aim to "filter" popular information, ensuring transmission of basic knowledge, seems obvious. Education will enable patients to prepare their general attitude regarding the use of novel applications with valid information, facilitating the role of attending physicians during the informed consent process. The patient organizations are major players in developing programs of education, along with medical associations, and official scientific media open to patient access.

Enhancement

The quality of patient information seems much more important, if perspectives of 3D bioprinting also include potential production and use of tissue and organs for enhancement purposes.[22] Indeed the method does not exclude that possibility, even with the intention to create novel biological material, not existing in Nature, with special characteristics.[23] The fact that the aim of use will be not to repair a certain pathological condition of the receiver, but to "improve" a healthy condition of the organism, changes substantially the role of attending physicians in the informed consent process.

In principle, anyone has a right to enhancement as an expression of self-determination and on condition that this does not affect other persons' rights.[24] Yet insofar enhancement presupposes an interventional medical act, physicians should be fully aware of potential risks that may occur for the healthy organism of the person interested. This does not only intensify their obligation to provide accurate and detailed information to the latter, stressing in particular the possibility of risks, but moreover it obliges them to check the general ability of the person involved in understanding the seriousness of such an intervention. This additional duty emerges from the fact that, generally speaking, rational reasoning is unfamiliar with medical interventions that may destabilize a healthy human organism.

Cell donors' data processing

The collection and use of cells for bioprinting purposes involves the issue of the donors' data protection.

The moral idea of data protection, in general, is that of the so-called "informational self-determination."[25] That notion suggests the acceptance of an intimate core in individual personality that needs to remain always under the direct control of its subject. As a dimension of the individual privacy, this core is composed by personal information (personal data), permitting the detection of a person's identity.

Most of personal data are "simple" in the sense that, if revealed, they do not have any significant further potential impact for their subject, besides identification. But there is also a category of the so-called "sensitive" data, which may have such significant impact involving risks for the subject's personal and social life. These are data concerning, for example, race, national origin, religious, philosophical and political beliefs, sexual orientation, sexual life, etc. Par excellence, sensitive data are those concerning the individual health or biological condition, including medical and biological data (biometric data, genetic data). Medical and biological data need, thus, specific protection, as their uncontrolled disclosure may affect substantially their subject's life, by triggering negative discriminations, in work, insurance, education, or by creating serious troubles in private life, family and sexual relations, etc.[26]

To avoid such implications, strict measures ensuring personal direct control particularly in medical and biological data, need to be considered. This is a legal issue, which attracts attention worldwide, nowadays, due to the development of informatics and the subsequent possibilities to collect, process, and transfer data. Yet the major ethical problem that we are facing, regarding the handling of biological data, springs from their importance for research purposes. The collection and processing of biological and particularly of genetic data are necessary for running research projects intending to the development of new diagnostic or therapeutic means, either drugs or medical devices and tools or even products for clinical use, including bioprinted transplant material.

In that perspective, the idea of data protection, involving a requirement for direct personal control of the data by the individual concerned, gives the impression of an obstacle. In other words, the necessity for data protection, serving their individual subject, potentially contravenes their value for research purposes, which may be beneficial for society as a whole. A generally accepted ethical maxim, according to which the interests of an individual always prevail over the interests of society, provides a rough normative framework for seeking a certain balance, but certainly a more detailed elaboration in relevance is needed.

This problem is crucial for bioprinting insofar the development of future clinical applications needs more research to achieve reliable results. To overcome risks for unwanted leakage of sensitive data without undermining research strategies, the best solution is that of the use of anonymous biological material, from nonidentifiable donors, at least at the basic research stage. In clinical research, though, identifiable material will be necessary, to check suitability in transplantations, therefore all strict guarantees for the protection of the donors' sensitive data need to be in place. Specific informed consent of the donor for reproducing the original material is the basic requirement, here, along with measures ensuring confidentiality in relevant data processing.

Reproductive material

A futuristic perspective for 3 D bioprinting includes the possibility to replicate reproductive material, particularly embryonic cell lines or even early embryos.[27]

The use of reproductive material, in general, presupposes also specific informed consent by the donors. In the case of embryonic material, both donors need to provide consent. Donors' data protection is also an issue, as gametes are biological material with the donor's genetic identity, and embryos share part of their genetic identity with both genitors. Therefore, all the aforementioned guarantees for the sensitive data protection need to be considered here, as well.

Bioprinting could be an option to overcome problems in availability of reproductive material, of ova in particular. Nowadays, limited availability of ova impedes seriously the access of many couples in assisted reproduction. The rule of donor anonymity (to ensure protection of privacy) has been abandoned in several countries, in an effort for encouraging personal donation of ova between relatives and friends.[28] On the other hand, the problem feeds a growing black market of ova (and, thus, women) trafficking worldwide.[29] A future perspective of using available ova in order to create early embryos with the purpose to extract totipotent stem cells as the original material for bioprinting, possibly provides a solution there.

Still, from an ethical point of view, specific consent of early embryos' genitors for bioprinting purposes will remain an undeniable prerequisite, even if the method could address such problems, because, any deliberate processing of original reproductive material by the clinic, intending to the use of replicated embryos by third persons, once again involves the issue of sensitive data protection, as this is identifiable material. That means that even surplus original reproductive material (surplus embryos) remains under the direct control of the donors and is not considered as "leftover" at the free disposal of the clinic.

Potential bioprinting of embryonic totipotent stem cell lines, in the future, could raise more serious ethical problems, in the sense that these blastocyst cells can be developed into complete human organism, following the full reproductive process. The question, here, is similar to the one discussed extensively with regard to possible future application of reproductive cloning in humans.

Indeed, bioprinted totipotent stem cell lines will have identical genetic profile with the original ones, leading to identical organisms, just like the clones. A basic objection to the creation of human clones suggests that the fact of creating intentionally identical twins undermines their human dignity, in the sense that these persons would be obliged to bear a lifelong burden to demonstrate uniqueness of their personality unlike their "designing."[30] Similar argumentation is valid for bioprinting also, as only the method of reproducing identical human beings, and not the intention as such, changes. Yet this is the only reason to reject human stem cell line bioprinting on ethical grounds. In contrast, as in the case of "therapeutic cloning," bioprinting stem cells just for developing transplant material does not present such ethical concerns, as no intention of creating identical human beings is involved.[31]

Access

Access to natural biological material for therapeutic purposes is a major issue in the context of transplantations. Due to the lack of reliable alternatives, systems ensuring equal access of patients to the extremely limited resource of available organs, based upon objective criteria of prioritization, are necessary even in advanced health systems.

Assuming that bioprinting could provide eventually such an alternative, with the use of original cells from the patient's organism, it seems that we can overcome the above problem of justice. Still access is not ensured if, in financial terms, 3D bioprinting is not affordable by the national health systems.[32] This is related to the more general problem of public funds' allocation in healthcare, but certainly the eligibility of 3D bioprinting for public funding should take into account its cost-efficiency in comparison with the current transplantation system's needs for funding.

Two elements seem to be crucial for relevant decision making. First, the degree in which we can confirm that the bioprinting alternative to conventional grafts is safe and functional for the patients, in order to determine comparative cost-efficiency. Second, a system of prioritizing patients, according to their therapeutic needs, in case where bioprinting is considered financially affordable by the public health systems, only for a partial coverage of potential receivers. That system will be similar to the one we already accept in transplantations, with the establishment of priority lists on conditions of fair access and transparency.

Regulation and law

Currently no specific legislation on 3D printing and bioprinting exists at the level of international or national law. Nevertheless, during the last three decades, legislation regulating in detail almost every major area of Biomedicine has been adopted worldwide. In addition, case-law addressed by the courts at various levels of jurisdiction (including constitutional and supreme national courts in most countries, as well as international courts, such as the European Court on Human Rights) produced an important part of regulation, covering difficult issues of the existing rules' interpretation. That corpus of legal regulation needs to be taken into consideration when discussing practical aspects regarding the application of novel biomedical methods and products, including, of course, the development and use of 3D printing and bioprinting.

The major reason justifying the role of legislation in Biomedicine is for ensuring certainty when novel technologies are to be applied. This means that we need to balance in a fair way all legitimate interests that, potentially, may be in conflict, of the persons involved (the patients, the doctors, the investigators, etc.). These interests express a variety of legal rights that need to be regulated accordingly. Most of these rights are fundamental, being established by constitutional or international rules; they are known as "human rights," and they prevail over other "common" rights. International legal instruments, such as the UN's Universal Declaration on Human Rights and the European Convention on Human Rights, are the basic references for the content of these rights. Relatively recent instruments, particularly the Council of Europe Convention on Human Rights and Biomedicine (Oviedo Convention) and the UNESCO's Universal Declaration on Human Rights and Bioethics indicate the relevance of human rights with topics of Medicine and Biomedicine, especially with applications of advanced technologies in Medicine.

In Europe, more specific legislation of the EU establishes detailed rules with binding force for the member states, including rules on data protection,[33] on clinical trials,[34] or on patenting in biotechnology.[35] The corpus of binding law in Europe, thus, contains, on the one hand, the Oviedo Convention's system (the Convention and its additional Protocols on Human Cloning, on Transplantations, on Biomedical Research, and on Genetic Testing for Health Purposes) and the aforementioned EU legislation. On the other hand, a significant piece of regulation springs from the relevant to Biomedicine case-law of the European Court on Human Rights[36] and of the EU's European Court of Justice.[37]

Although the issues emerging from biomedical innovations need to be addressed ethically in a consistent way, under common universal principles, the respective legal reflection should always refer to concrete binding rules and their determined force within certain geographical area, with the exception of very few instruments of international law, universally accepted. In the following, thus, we will investigate the legal dimension of 3D printing and bioprinting in the framework of the European law, as defined previously. This does not mean, of course, that a legal approach based upon the US (or other western type) law cannot lead to similar legal conclusions.

Clinical trials

In European Biolaw, the standard legal framework for the regulation of clinical research is that of the Oviedo Convention system. Inspired by the nonlegal codes of ethics in relevance (particularly, that of the Helsinki Declaration[38]), the Convention itself encompasses a chapter regarding clinical research, declaring the fundamental legal principles for the protection of persons undergoing research.[39] The Additional Protocol on Biomedical Research of the Convention develops in detail these principles. At the EU level, specific legislation exists only for interventional clinical studies (clinical trials) on pharmaceutical products, which is actually the most important part of applied clinical research.[40] For 3D printing and bioprinting, thus, only the Oviedo Convention system is relevant, and only for the countries that have already accepted (ratified) its instruments.[41]

According to the principles of that system, printed devices, implants, or biological material may be tested in patients, only when (1) no alternative with comparable effectiveness exists, (2) potential risks for the person involved are not disproportionate if compared with the benefits expected, (3) previous appropriate approval of the research protocol by competent scientific and ethics bodies has been obtained, (4) patients involved have already been informed about their rights and guarantees, provided by law, and (5) the necessary patient informed consent has been given previously, in explicit, specific and documented form, and can be withdrawn at any time. In addition, when patients to be involved are persons unable to provide appropriate consent (minors, or adults with mental or cognitive disabilities), more strict guarantees are applied, namely (1) expected benefits for health should be direct and real, (2) no alternative to perform research with persons able to provide consent exists, (3) a written and specific permission has been provided by the legal representative of the person involved (who is responsible, in general, to provide informed consent), and (4) the patient involved does not object to the research.

Supposing that the safety issues for the use of printed material have been addressed successfully in preclinical animal studies, we need to imagine the particular circumstances for its experimental use in humans under the abovementioned legal prerequisites. Two relevant issues should be noticed in this respect.

First, alternatives to the use of bioprinted material in particular could be only confirmed methods of natural biological material use (standard cell therapies, or other methods of regenerative Medicine, approved by competent official bodies).

Yet a certain method of cell therapy (with genuine cells) may also be at an experimental stage. In that case, the same principles need to be considered for that method as well. If no approved alternative exists, we need to make a choice between the two experimental methods, that of the bioprinted material, and that of the genuine material. The law does not provide an explicit answer, in such a case, so the attending physician must judge according to the best interest of the patient, that is, according to the risk/benefit comparing evaluation of both options. This evaluation is necessary, even when the bioprinted option meets the second prerequisite on risk/benefit evaluation (proportionate risks) if examined as a sole option.

The second issue is that of the implementation in practice of the patient's right to withdraw.[42] To reject the use of bioprinted material as a therapeutic strategy, after entering the study, means that the patient wishes to restore his/her condition of health before incorporating the printed material. The question, here, is whether transplanted biological material produces reversible effects to the organism or not.

Withdrawal of patients in the setting of clinical trials for medicinal products (drugs) means that the patient does not receive any more the substance to be tested. Even if the previous administration of that substance has produced certain effects to the patient's organism, such effects will stop at some time after withdrawal, which means that restoration is feasible. This is not the case with transplanted tissue or organs, as any restoration presupposes new operation with the relevant risks. Therefore, the right to withdraw means a certain burden for the patient; it cannot be exercised without a risk/benefit appraisal. In any case, the physician's responsibility is more intense there, due to this weak status of a legitimate option that patients' normally enjoy.

Transplantations

The clinical use of bioprinted tissue (or, possibly, solid organs) in the future involves also the law for transplantations. In Europe, the additional Protocol on Transplantations of the Oviedo Convention (2002) provides the basic regulation in relevance. Also, for the EU member states a Directive regarding the safe storage and handling of biological material (but not of solid organs) purposing for clinical use should also be considered.[43]

The aim of the Protocol is to provide standards of protection for the respective rights of both the donors and receivers (patients), given the limited availability of tissue and organs which is the major problem in transplantations worldwide. Since the basis of that regulation is a need for the use of third persons' biological material, the option of 3D bioprinting seems to overcome drastically that problem. By reproducing original tissue from the patient, self-transplantation operations will cover a big part of the current graft demand. In that respect, no necessity for ensuring donors' and receivers' rights, according to the current legal framework exists. Still, as far as graft safety and functioning issues are persistent, in the sense that the quality of bioprinted grafts compared to the natural available grafts remains unconfirmed, the enforcement of rights in transplantations will be an issue. That means, also, that distribution of organs, according to the prioritization of patients following legally established criteria, will not be affected, until the bioprinting alternative provides evidence of equal quality for replacing natural grafts.

On the other hand, on the assumption that the original biological material to be printed is not part of the patient's organism, but obtained by another person, a question is whether the same guarantees for the protection of that person's rights are in place, as in the case of conventional tissue and organ donation from living donors.[44] Even if with bioprinting we can overcome current limits in reproducing biological material for clinical purposes, the fact that the original material has been removed from a natural human organism raises all known problems regarding safety and protection of the donor autonomy. Again, these problems should be treated in accordance with the Protocol, as in conventional transplantations.

Human reproduction

In Europe, assisted reproduction is governed currently by national legislations.[45] Common European legal provisions are very few.[46] Also the case-law of the European Court on Human Rights accepts a large margin of appreciation for the national legislator to regulate fertility issues, abstaining from acknowledging common rules in relevance.[47]

Nevertheless, the additional Protocol of the Oviedo Convention, prohibiting cloning in humans, could also be applied in regard to future bioprinting applications with the use of human embryos. It is true that, in its preamble, the Protocol is referred explicitly to cloning in its technical meaning,[48] but still the rational to avoid reproduction of identical human beings stands, even when similar to cloning techniques drive to the same result. The wording of the article 1 of the Protocol supports also this interpretation, by making reference to the prohibition of "any intervention" ("seeking to create a human being genetically identical to another human being").

Another issue related to the application of bioprinting methodology on early embryos could be its compliance with the legal regulation of research in embryos in vitro, according to the Oviedo Convention. The relevant article 18 poses two rules on that matter: (1) research in embryos in vitro is allowed only if "adequate protection" of the embryo is ensured, and (2) the creation of embryos just for research purposes is prohibited.

The hypothetical scenario of embryo bioprinting involves the application of both rules. On the one hand, the original material would be embryos in vitro, created artificially for reproductive purposes in the first place. According to the first rule of article 18, these embryos should be "protected" if used for bioprinting, that is, their developmental potential needs to be maintained. On the other hand, the second rule of article 18 seems to impede the creation of replicated embryos, if research is the original purpose, allowing bioprinting only if there is scientific evidence that these embryos could follow a normal developmental process, meaning that they may serve reproductive purposes.

It is obvious that, as far as lack of sufficient evidence exists, requiring more research on replicated embryos (therefore no reproductive use is possible), that normative impediment bans even basic research on 3D bioprinting with early embryos, under the Oviedo Convention system.

Data protection

The new legislation in the EU on data protection (the General Data Protection Regulation—GDPR), compared to the previous regulation of Directive 95/46, introduces a substantial change regarding the use of personal data for research purposes. According to the new Regulation, the previously required specific nature of the subject's consent has been replaced by a less strict concept of consent pertaining not exclusively to the concrete research project but intending to cover also potential use of data for future research activities in the broader area of scientific interest.[49]

That change in regulation certainly facilitates research initiatives in Biomedicine, by taking, however, risks concerning the protection of patient data, since data collection and flow are allowed under easier conditions. Focusing on 3D bioprinting and given the need for developing extensive research before reaching an acceptable level of safety and functional suitability for the clinical use of bioprinted tissues and organs, this new regulatory environment requires a careful approach. It is worth noting that, generally speaking, facilitation of procedures does not necessarily create legal certainty when rules are to be applied in concrete situations. For instance, the fact that no previous license by the DP Authority is required reduces legal certainty and increases the risk of exposure to legal sanctions,[50] since the burden of compliance with the relevant rules is transferred to the research team with no previous official notification about the details of compliance. In the past, compliance was ensured by the licensing system; it is now up to the research units' legal advisors and data protection officers[51] to play that role, but with no official guarantee on data protection best practices.

In contrast, the change in the concept of the data subjects' consent is not expected to create problems in legal certainty. There is no question that identifiable medical data will be necessary for testing the research results in bioprinting, which means that the consent requirement lies on the core of research procedures. At first glance, even under the previous regime of specific consent, research would not be impeded, since the original cells are intended to be processed for specific purpose (the production of bioprinted tissue or organ), which could be explained in detail to the donor (and subject of data) prior to provide consent. Under the current regime of "broad" consent, the same material could also be used for similar research projects in bioprinting, not necessarily after being described in their details to the donor during the information process. It is sufficient to inform the donor about that potential use by determining only the field of research in general terms, that is, "bioprinting." Legally, that practice would be in absolute compliance with the GDPR framework.

Commercialization

A further legal question concerns potential commercialization of bioprinted tissue and organs. Commercialization is discussed as an incentive for promoting research in bioprinting by attracting investments at an industrial scale, with the expectation of profit. Of course, the option of autologous transplantations[52] with the use of bioprinted grafts emanated from biological material of the patient/receiver does not concern organ marketing. But the perspective of the embryonic stem cell use, as original material for producing bioprinted tissue and organs, leaves the question of commercial exploitation open.

According to the article 22 of the Oviedo Convention, and the articles 21, 22 of its additional Protocol on Transplantations, commercialization of the human body and its parts is explicitly prohibited. The question, thus, is whether we can consider bioprinted organs as "parts of the human body," firstly because they would be products of the processing of original human biological material, and, secondly, because they are supposed to be perfectly functional in the human organism, if transplanted.

Article 22 addresses the problem of potential organ trafficking for transplantation use, in conditions of scarcity of that valuable resource worldwide, by adopting a strict policy that rejects the commodification of human organs. Since no idea about 3D bioprinting and its potential to produce organs existed at the time of the Convention's promulgation, one could argue that article 22 refers only to natural "parts of the body" and not to artificial products of tissue engineering or bioprinting. According to this approach, commodification and commercialization of bioprinted organs would be legally allowed. Yet a counterargument could raise an issue about commodification as such, as violating the principle of human dignity (article 1 of the Convention[53]). Since bioprinted organs emanated from the processing of human biological material, they can be considered as an "extension" of the latter, sharing a common expression of human dignity which excludes commodification. In other words, the prohibition stated by article 22 is not justified on the grounds of a certain policy (combating organ trafficking), but on the grounds of human dignity, as a fundamental ethical and legal principle; that principle denies any instrumentalization of the human body[54] and its parts, a characteristic example of which is commodification.

The identification of bioprinted organs in terms of the ethical and legal status of the original biological material is questionable. These organs would be rather "products" and not "parts" of the human body, as they are the result of an artificial process. In that sense, they do not "contribute" to the status of dignity of any particular person, as they did not even exist as parts of a certain human body. Therefore, in that case, the notion of instrumentalization is meaningless; no person is affected by the production and use of bioprinted organs, at least prior to their transplantation for therapeutic purposes. In reality, this argumentation fits also all methods of human tissue engineering, in general, leaving the option of commercial exploitation legally acceptable.

Conclusions

Ethical considerations, regarding 3D printing of devices, implants, or other nonbiological objects useful for medical purposes are mostly related to safety and informed consent issues, both in experimental procedures (clinical trials) and in therapeutic settings.

Safety is always relative, since certain vigilance is, not only scientifically but also ethically, required even after the successful concluding of trials, in order to detect in the long-run side effects to the patients' organism from the use of these objects. Accurate information of patients about the details of such a use is equally important, as misunderstandings about the real expectations for their therapeutic advantages may occur, due to the general information that patients receive from unreliable but popular sources. This problem is even more serious in the case of bioprinting.

There is no doubt that 3D bioprinting represents a new era in regenerative medicine, as it makes possible the production of human tissue and organs at a large scale, already developed as a real industrial activity.[55] Scarcity in biological material for transplantations is currently the major obstacle in the development of regenerative medicine, and 3D bioprinting seems to be a convincing option to address that problem. As a new method, thus, bioprinting is expected to open enormous possibilities in medical treatment, which means that, in terms of its objective, its ethical value is unquestionable.

Nevertheless, several ethical and legal issues associated mostly to the methodology both in research and clinical use need thorough investigation. As for the first time we are facing the possibility to create functional human material, elaborated artificially, to provide a reliable alternative for natural grafts in transplantations, a common perception is that our technology is now able to produce parts of the human body without the need of the whole body! Should we acknowledge a certain ethical status to these entities or, to be more precise, should we respect certain ethical limitations in their use? This is a fundamental question, of a rather philosophical nature though.

But there are also more practical questions, regarding the acceptable level of safety for clinical use, the conditions of clinical research with regard to the patients' rights and interests, the data protection issue even in basic research, the potential for replicating early embryos, and the problem of fair access for all patients.

Such questions are also conceptualized in a legal framework, not yet specific for bioprinting, but still highly relevant, as the progress of Biolaw during the last decades tends to cover in detail similar issues emerged in transplantations, clinical trials, patient/doctor relationships, embryo research, etc. The European law, in particular, is characterized by legislative initiatives, intending to supranational binding regulation, working thus on the general legal framework rather than on specific cases. This ensures certainty in regulation, on condition of a continuous monitoring its efficacy and permanent updating. In general, one can conclude that legal solutions regarding the questions that occurred in bioprinting are feasible even under the current legal framework in Europe. These solutions are not necessarily in favor of relevant research and clinical use, but still they indicate issues needing a fresh approach, possibly demanding legislative amendments.

After several decades of impressive technological progress, triggering intensive ethical and legal reflection, we understand that the important in biomedical innovations, is to demonstrate real benefits for individual patients specifically, and for the healthcare system as a whole. The approach of ethics and law should promote this process, by expressing a practical attitude. This is the case of 3D printing and bioprinting as well, even if its products seem still alien (and perhaps scary) for the common people.

Endnotes

1. Al Ali AB, Griffin MF, Butler PE. Three-dimensional printing surgical applications. Eplasty 2015; 15:352—67.
2. Li J, Chen M, Fan X, Zhou H. Recent advances in bioprinting techniques: approaches, applications and future prospects. J Transl Med 2016;14. Passim Murphy SV, Atala A. 3D bioprinting of tissues and organs. Nat Biotechnol 2014;32(8); passim.
3. Al Ali et al., 357.
4. Al Ali et al., 353.
5. See art. Two of the Council of Europe's Convention on Human Rights and Biomedicine (1997).
6. Patuzzo S, Goracci G, Ciliberti R, Gasperini L. 3D bioprinting technology: scientific aspects and ethical issues. Sci Eng Ethics 2017;10; Gilbert F, Viana JNM, O'Connell CD, Dodds S. Enthusiastic portrayal of 3D bioprinting in the media: ethical side effects. Bioethics 2017;6—7.
7. WHO/The Uppsala Monitoring Center, The importance of Pharmacovigilance. Safety monitoring of medicinal products, WHO ed. 2002, Chapt. 4.
8. See, in general, Andorno R. The precautionary principle: a new legal standard for a technological age. J Int Biotech L 2004;1:11. Also, in the field of "soft-law," see The Rio Declaration on Environment and Development (Rio de Janeiro, 1992), Principle 15.
9. For other moral dilemmas in relevance, see Caplan AL. Is xenografting morally wrong? (Transplantation Proceedings 1992). In: Kuhse H, Singer P, editor. Bioethics. An anthology. Oxford: Blackwell; 1999, p. 404.
10. See, for the Nazi's Germany and Japan's experience, McNeill PM. Experimentation on human beings. In: Kuhse H, Singer P, editors. A companion to bioethics. Oxford: Blackwell; 2001, p. 369. Also, in the U.S., Curran WJ. The Tuskagee syphilis study. N Eng J Med 1973;730.
11. Beauchamp TL, Childress JF. Principles of biomedical ethics, fifth ed. Oxford U.P.; 2001. p. 77.
12. See, in that line, Patuzzo S, et al. p. 10.
13. Beauchamp TL, Childress JF. p. 38.
14. Cantor NL. A patient's decision to decline life-saving medical treatment: bodily integrity versus the preservation of life. Rut L Rev 1973;26:228—64.
15. See Moskop JC, Iserson KV. Triage in medicine, part II: underlying values and principles. Ann Emerg Med 2007;49:282—7, Oviedo Convention, article 8.
16. Capron AM. Advance directives. In: Kuhse H, Singer P, editors. A companion to bioethics. Oxford: Blackwell; 2001. p. 261.
17. See, in general, Beauchamp TL, Childress JF. pp. 88—93.
18. Beauchamp TL, Childress JF. p. 83.
19. Beauchamp TL, Childress JF. p. 95.
20. Gilbert F, et al. p. 1.
21. For the responsibility of experts regarding the presentation of scientific announcements to the public, see Gilbert F, et al. p. 9.

22. See Patuzzo S, et al. pp. 5—7.
23. Ozbolat I, Peng W, Ozbolat V. Application areas of 3 D bioprinting. Drug Discov Today 2016;12.
24. As it happens, for instance, with the doping use in competitive environments (sports, education).
25. Rouvroy A, Poullet Y. The right to informational self-determination and the value of self-development: reassessing the importance of privacy in democracy. In: Gurwirth S, et al., editors. Reinventing data protection? Springer, Science+Business Media B.V.; 2009. p. 45.
26. See, for example, European Group on Ethics, Ethical Aspects of Genetic Testing in the Workplace, Opinion No 18, Brussels; 2003. Low L, King S, Wilkie T. Genetic discrimination in life insurance: empirical evidence from a cross sectional survey of genetic support groups in the United Kingdom. BMJ 1998;317:1632—5.
27. The creation of hybrids by mingling human and animal reproductive material is also discussed, in ethics terms, although explicitly prohibited in several national legislations. See, in relevance, Patuzzo S, et al. p. 8.
28. See on that question, Nelson MK, Hertz R, Kramer W. Gamete donor anonymity and limits on numbers of offspring: the views of three stakeholders J L Biosci 2016;3:39—67.
29. Deveaux M. Exploitation, structural injustice, and the cross-border trade in human ova. J Global Ethics 2016;12(1):48—68.
30. See, in that line, Habermas J. The future of human nature. Cambridge, UK:Polity; 2003. p. 42, 63, 78.
31. Still, there are strong religious beliefs objecting to the use of embryos in general, considering the ethical status of embryos equal to the status of a person. See Patuzzo S, et al. p. 7.
32. According to an argument, the access of some people that can afford that cost might encourage general access. See Patuzzo S, et al. p. 11.
33. General Data Protection Regulation 679/2016.
34. Clinical Trial Regulation 536/2014 (its implementation is still pending).
35. Directive 98/44.
36. Particularly on patient/physician relationships, assisted suicide, and assisted reproduction.
37. Particularly on patents in biological applications (in relevance with the breast cancer genes BRCA 1, 2, and the processing of embryonic stem cells).
38. The WMA's Helsinki Declaration (*Ethical Principles for Medical Research Involving Human Subjects*—1964/2013) is the most famous nonlegal instrument on clinical research, which inspired the relevant international or national legal instruments.
39. Chapter V (art. 15—17).
40. Directives 2001/20, 2005/28, still in force, but to be replaced after the implementation of the Clinical Trial Regulation. See, in detail: https://www.ema.europa.eu/en/human-regulatory/research-development/clinical-trials/clinical-trial-regulation.
41. See the relevant list of the Council of Europe's member states in: https://rm.coe.int/inf-2017-7-rev-etat-sign-ratif-reserves/168077dd22.
42. See art. 16 v.
43. Directive 2004/23.
44. See Protocol, Chapter III (art. 9—15).
45. In most countries, including the UK, France, Spain, Italy, Greece, etc.
46. See, especially, the article 14 of the Oviedo Convention, on prohibition of embryo sex selection.
47. See, for example, *Paradiso and Campanelli v. Italy* [GC] - 25,358/12 Judgment 24.1.2017 [GC].
48. By making reference to "embryo splitting" and "nuclear transfer."
49. See para 33 of the preamble.
50. For the sanctions, see articles 83, 84 of the GDPR.
51. See in relevance, articles 37—39 GDPR.
52. S. Murphy, A. Atala, 781.
53. "Parties to this Convention shall protect the dignity and identity of all human beings and guarantee everyone, without discrimination, respect for their integrity and other rights and fundamental freedoms with regard to the application of biology and medicine."

54. See, in general, Schmidt H. Whose dignity? Resolving ambiguities in the scope of "human dignity" in the Universal Declaration on Bioethics and Human Rights. J Med Ethics 2007;33:579.

55. BIS Research. Global bioprinting market-analysis and forecast, 2018–2025, Fremont CA; 2018. In: https://bisresearch.com/industry-report/global-bioprinting-market-2025.html.

Quality and safety in medical 3D printing

5

Georgios Georgantis, MD, PhD [1], **Evanthia Kostidi, PhD** [2], **Ioannis Dagkinis, PhD** [2],
Dimitrios Papachristos, PhD [3], **Nikitas Nikitakos** [4]

[1]*Academic Fellow, Aristotle University of Thessaloniki, Thessaloniki, Greece;* [2]*Department of Shipping Trade & Transport, University of the Aegean, Chios, Greece;* [3]*University of West Attica, Greece;* [4]*Professor, Department of Shipping Trade & Transport, University of the Aegean, Chios, Greece*

Introduction

The AM/3DP (additive manufacturing/3D printing) is a type of manufacturing technique wherein the final object is formed by successive addition of layers of materials such as plastics, metals, drugs, cell culture etc. using the 3D printer (see Fig. 5.1) [1]. According to United States Governmental Accountability Office (GAO), 3D printing can create 3D structures from digital models by AM process [2]. It has a wide

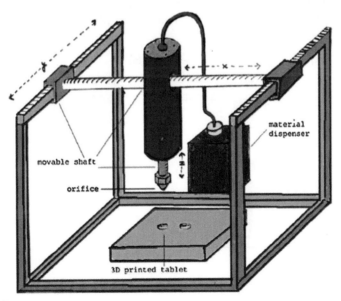

FIGURE 5.1

3D printer with different components [6].

3D Printing: Applications in Medicine and Surgery. https://doi.org/10.1016/B978-0-323-66164-5.00005-2
Copyright © 2020 Elsevier Inc. All rights reserved.

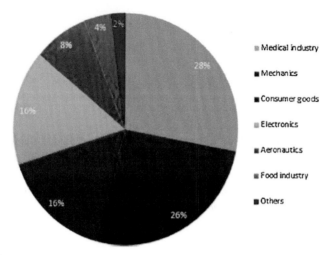

FIGURE 5.2

Pie chart showing applications of 3D printing in various fields [6].

range of applications in various fields including healthcare, automobile, aerospace, food, chemical, and toy industry (see Fig. 5.2). In the healthcare industry, 3D printing has been used to produce various dosage forms of drugs, prosthetics, medical devices, and artificial tissues and organs. 3D bioprinting is the fabrication of a functional artificial tissues or organs via a 3D printer such as Regenova [2] by layer-upon-layer addition of cells, biomaterials [3] using bioinks such as

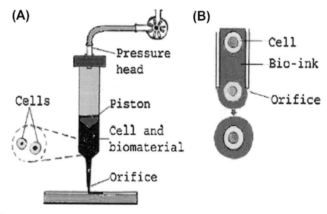

FIGURE 5.3

Pictorial representation of bioprinter. (A) Bioprinter and (B) printer head [6].

endotoxin-free low-acyl gellan gum [4](see Fig. 5.3). For example, Spritam,[a] the first 3D-printed drug approved by FDA has encouraged tremendous research in the development of various medication by the use of 3D printing technology [5]. This innovation comes with various challenges to be looked upon to combat the disruptions that can possibly occur ([6], p. 146).

Various disruptions in healthcare and manufacturing due to 3D printing are predicted to occur. For more than 20 years, applications of 3D printing were restricted to prototyping. In the recent years, many of the 3D-printed objects have been introduced in the market of healthcare and manufacturing such as medical devices (prosthetics), dental instruments (crowns, bridges), artificial organs (kidney, heart) for research purposes, implants, and many others. By 2019, 3D-printed objects will be a part of our daily life, "located" in or on the body of more than 10% people in the developed world. 3D printing will play a crucial role in more than 35% of the surgical procedures requiring prosthetics, implants, artificial organs, and other 3D-printed objects. Advancement in technology and innovations will lead to 10% of spurious drugs and pharmaceuticals manufactured using 3D printer [7].

3D printing can increase the quality of deliverable healthcare services, as it is capable of manufacturing personalized products suited for a particular individual. It can print medicine in various shapes, sizes, doses, and dosage forms with desired and prespecified characteristics, including drug release profile and fixed dose combination (FDC). Formulations prepared in an individualized manner are likely to increase drug safety and reduce toxicity and various other side effects caused by inappropriate drug dose. Likewise, the ability of 3D printers to fabricate the medicine at the point-of-care (PoC) avails a range of therapeutic options, which removes the barrier for healthcare personnel in choosing the best-suited approach. Further, it is capable of producing various medical devices, implants, anatomical models, artificial organs, among others, covering a large potential for overall betterment of healthcare services and healthcare education. The first FDA-approved drug product demonstrated the commercial applicability of 3D-printed products in August 2015 following which a large number of medical devices have been produced via 3D printing. Therefore, the continuous innovation and developments in 3D printing technique and its applications seem promising in terms of revolutionizing healthcare and improving quality of life ([6], p. 151).

Since 1993, continuous assessment of the process on a detailed basis has been carried out by disclosing some of the limitations in the new technology. Biomedical 3D printing nowadays not only has major applications in pharmaceutics, medicine, and dentistry, but it also involves strict regulation and social challenges. Legislation has to be adapted in order to characterize the new terminology of the new technology. Furthermore, issues like 3D data ownership, privacy and the protection of intellectual property rights must be faced. Quality and Safety standards also must be addressed, to ensure the well-being of humans. On the other hand, the use of the

---

[a] Levetiracetam, an antiepileptic drug.

new technology, the high offer of new materials and the technology itself is indisputably extremely challenging for various reasons. For instance, transplantation of a 3D-printed organ would be most welcome, given the lack of suitable donors. Lastly, there is always the prospect of new technology (high-end) new jobs ([6], pp. 147−152).

Quality assurance in medical 3D printing

In recent years the development of relatively cheap desktop 3D printers has led to a booming 3D printing industry. Now, with the arrival of commercially available biocompatible and sterilizable 3D prints, local medical 3D printing labs emerge in hospitals worldwide [8]. Studies show that medical 3D printing can be in many different ways of great added value for all kind of specializations. Three main applications are defined [9]:

- **Anatomic models**: The added value of 3D-printed anatomical models is threefold:
  - a valuable tool for physicians in patient−doctor communication [10,11];
  - serve as a tool for resident education and surgical training [12]; and
  - allow development for optimal surgical planning [13].

Furthermore, the quality of the preoperative plans based on 3D prints is shown to be higher than that of digital 3D-rendered images [14].

- **Surgical models**: 3D-printed surgical guides are widely used in specialties such as orthopedics, traumatology, oral and maxillofacial surgery, plastic surgery, and several other invasive surgical fields. Patient-specific surgical navigation guides offer a boost in surgical precision and reduction of surgical time, leading to lesser chance for infection and a faster recovery [15,16].
- **Implants and prostheses**: Development of implants and personalized prostheses is the most important and most valuable application of 3D printing in the field of orthopedics, up to now. Several individual cases of 3D-printed cranial, dental, and spinal implants have been reported [17].

With this rapidly growing new in-hospital technology, there's an urge and necessity for methods of quality control and quality assurance. Apart from a recent paper from Ref. [18]; where a methodology is provided for quality control of the in-house 3D printing workflow for unsterilized anatomical models, no literature on the quality control of the complete process, encompassing the various applications, is known. During the different phases of 3D printing, there is the possibility of errors occurring. These errors may be due to human factors such as miscommunication or failure of other factors which are inherent to the workflow step. By optimizing the workflow and a proper definition of the responsibilities, the human errors can be minimized or completely taken away, whereas the inherent errors can only be minimized and monitored. Specifically ([19], pp. 670−672),

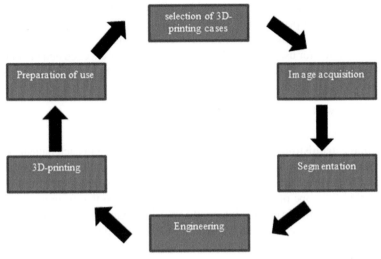

FIGURE 5.4

The 3D printing workflow [19].

1. *Qualitatively induced errors*: Without a well-defined 3D printing workflow strategy, the quality of the 3D printing process cannot be assured. The process definition contains a typical 3D printing workflow with six steps (Fig. 5.4):
   a. the selection of 3D printing cases (based on the clinical value, cost-effectiveness, and a risk assessment),
   b. image acquisition (responsibility of the radiologist and medical physicist),
   c. segmentation (reconstructing images is a collaboration between a technologist with anatomical knowledge, the requesting physician, and a medical engineer),

Step	1. Selection	2. Scan	3. Segment	4. Engineer	5. Print	6. Prepare
Competence	Value/cost Risk analysis	Anatomy Pathology Technical Dosimetry	Anatomy Pathology Technical	Technical	Technical	Anatomy Technical
Responsibility	Physician Physicist	Radiologist Physicist Technologist	Technologist	Engineer Physician	Engineer	Engineer Physician CSSD

FIGURE 5.5

3D printing process definition with a definition of steps and distribution of responsibilities [19].

    d. engineering (development of molds or guides, the smoothing and the supporting of the printable),

    e. 3D printing (a task for the medical engineer), and

    f. preparation for use (supports by a medical engineer, checked and validated by the requesting physician and if necessary sterilized at the central sterile service department (CSSD)).

An overview of the process see the next figure (Fig. 5.5):

- *Quantitatively induced errors*: these concern the following:
  - **Image acquisition and segmentation:** A critical step in each patient specific 3D print is the image acquisition. As the commonly used imaging modalities already own a QC program the quality control of the image acquisition is left out of the scope of this report. However, it is evident that from patient to digital scan, this is the first inherently error-inducing step in the process. Slice thickness and reconstruction kernels are the most important parameters at this stage. The segmentation is called the process of restricting the reconstructed volumetric images into the region of interest only. Within each of these packages segmentation can be achieved through various methods (Hounsfield units to slice per slice contouring). For a successful quality assurance program these induced errors should be insightful and easily monitored over time.
  - **3D printing**: It is evident that from CAD drawing to 3D print, the 3D printer induces errors due to the discrete layers that build up the model. The printer's resolution and accuracy are the parameters that could lead to unexpected dimensional errors.
  - **Sterilization:** For several 3D printing purposes, sterilization of the finished product is necessary. Possibilities are surgical instruments, surgical guides, and implants. In high-temperature steam sterilization, the 3D print is exposed for 3 minutes to temperatures of 134 °C.[b] Today, it is unclear if significant shrinkage, expansion, or deterioration of the print occurs at these temperatures.

For example, a case study in 2009 by Sampat et al., suggested that the rapid release and absorption of a baclofen compounded formulation may lead to toxicities in the targeted populations and that a reduced frequency of dosing is a suitable alternative for improved therapeutic outcomes [20]. Therefore, a modified release pediatric formulation, enabling individualization of dosage, could be the most suitable strategy to improve the therapeutic outcome of baclofen, with minimal side effects in the targeted population. Scoutaris et al. [21]; reported the development of chewable indomethacin 3D printed tablets ("Starmix") for the pediatric population using HPMCAS [21]. However, there are limited/no reports on the use of PVA for the development of pediatric

---

[b] WIPrichtlijn, http://www.rivm.nl/dsresource?objectid=330dd0f8-e6b8-4621-86b17a039ac83d42&type=pdf&disposition=inline.

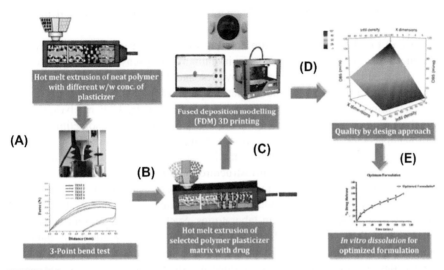

FIGURE 5.6

Diagram for the development of pediatric baclofen minicaplets; Point A: Hot melt extrusion of neat polymer and neat polymer with different concentrations of plasticizer; Point B: Three-point bend test was performed to characterize the polymeric blend with suitable elasticity; Point C: Hot melt extrusion of selected polymer-plasticizer matrix with drug was done; Point D: Minicaplets were designed and printed using a benchtop single nozzle FDM 3D printer; Point E: A quality of design approach was selected to optimize the formulation [22].

population-specific 3D-printed baclofen formulation. Thus, the purpose of the present work was to develop and characterize a modified release baclofen minicaplet using FDM 3D printing technique and systematically investigate the effect of different printing parameters on drug release using a 32 full factorial design. The overall process of hot melt extrusion to 3D printing of minicaplet and potential advantages of 3D-printed minicaplets in pediatric population have been schematically represented in the next figure ([22], pp. 107−108) (Fig. 5.6).

Safety in medical 3D printing

Safety constitutes a major regulatory challenge in the field of 3D printing. 3D printing is under constant influence from the development of new techniques and materials. This poses risks to safety in relation to the 3D printers, as well as the manufactured goods. In the domain of bioprinting, safety refers primarily to the risks associated with undertaking medical procedures outside professional medical environments. Safety issues include sources of biomaterials, unhealthy donors, implant efficacy, and posttransplant infections. 3D bioprinting remains an untested clinical paradigm and is based on the use of living cells placed into a human body; risks include teratoma and cancer, dislodgement and migration of implanted material ([23], p. 11).

Several bio-AM applications are entering the clinical trial phase, thereby also creating issues regarding safety testing in humans for disease modeling or testing of pharmaceuticals (e.g., 3D-printed ovaries and life-size printing of cartilage, bone, ear, muscle tissues, and biocompatible polymers) ([23], p. 11, [24]).

Other important safety issues concern the printing materials themselves, and the actual printing process. For instance, the use of novel polymers, sometimes mixed with nanoparticles, poses long-term risks for implants and requires postmarketing surveillance and registries. In addition, the increased level of customization and potential for more decentralization infrastructure may make it more difficult for consumers and authorities to verify the safety of products. Furthermore, higher safety standards apply for medical products other than consumer goods, and rules also govern the use of living tissues in laboratories. Such standards present barriers to personalized 3D-printed medical devices reaching the market. While these standards could change to support the development of "mass customization" for all kinds of medical devices, the changes will continue to prioritize patient safety and affect how a 3D printing infrastructure could emerge within the medical sector ([23], p. 12, [22]).

The location of manufacture matters in terms of establishing the compatibility of a 3D printing material with biological materials and the printing process. Specifically, a laboratory with controlled conditions and safety standards or a production plant with quality assurance practices in place Good Manufacturing Processes (GMP) differs from development and production at home. Cells and living tissues should be handled under strict safety procedures as in laboratories, to prevent distribution of, e.g., blood-borne diseases when patient material is used in manufacturing. Furthermore, 3D printing will make it possible to manufacture devices and products in a decentralized way ([23], p. 12, [22]).

For example, 3D bioprinting is a tool within the broader fields of tissue engineering and stem cell therapy. Many of the risks inherent in these fields will carry over to bioprinting (Vacanti and Langer 1999 [25–27]; see Table 5.1). As the complexity of the bioprinted tissues increases, the associated risks are multiplied ([28,29] see Table 5.2). This is especially apparent with the future possibility of bioprinting artificial organs (Murphy and Atala 2014, [26,30]; see Table 5.3).

Legal considerations for medical 3D printing

The use of AM (or 3D printing) in medicine, dentistry, and pharmaceutical sectors has created numerous legal considerations. Kritikos [23]. groups them into:

- Legal classification of 3D printing;
- Intellectual property rights;
- Data protection aspects;

Table 5.1 Risk of harms associated with tissue engineering [31].

Technology	Goal	Risks of harm to human
Tissue engineering	The aim of tissue engineering is to isolate living cells from small tissue samples, multiply them in the laboratory, and seed them onto biomaterial "scaffolds" that direct cell development toward functioning tissues for implantation	The implantation of any material in the body carries with it some risk that the body will recognize it as a foreign invader and engulf it with macrophages, resulting in inflammation. After implantation, possible defective tissues, teratoma, or the dislodgement and migration of implant materials and cells, are compounded by the fact that the implantation may be an irreversible process. Increases risk of harm to recipient because the degradation produces by-products which can then move through the bloodstream. The materials must be designed to pass through the renal system without harming the body. Risks associated with biodegradation by-products include cytotoxicity, clotting, inefficient excretion resulting in a build up of toxins in the body, and migration of by-products resulting in the disruption of another organ. Biomaterials derived from nonhuman organisms may carry their own risks, such as immunological responses and the risk of introducing pathogen. The use of living stem cells in any bioprinting therapy, even cells derived from the patient, carries risks, including tumor formation, immunological reactions, the unpredictable behavior of the cells, and long-term health effects yet unknown.

- Liability;
- Safety issues;
- Security; and
- Socioethical considerations.

In terms of the intellectual property, there are the morality clauses, that is 3D products/processes must pass the "morality acceptability test" in order to become

Table 5.2 Risk of harms associated with 3D bioprinting [31].

Technology	Goal	Risks of harm to human
3D bioprinting	Bioprinting process often involves extrusion of cells, encapsulated in a synthetic scaffold medium, through a narrow nozzle, subjecting them to high shear forces.	The transient forces may act to direct stem cells toward an undesired lineage.
	The bioprinting process requires a "bioink" medium that serves to carry the cells during printing and to encapsulate them in a 3D matrix after deposition.	3D bioprinting process often requires a curing step whereby the printed (liquid) bioink is transformed into a more solid form. This curing step often involves exposure to UV light and cross-linking initiation chemicals. Again, though the toxicity of curing is screened in the short term, the ultimate effects of such exposure may include DNA damage and may not be apparent until after implantation.
		The bioink materials are more likely to be synthetic (e.g., polyethylene glycol) or to be chemically modified natural materials.
		Also unique to bioprinting, the layer-by-layer printing process creates an inherent heterogeneity in the printed structure. This may generate "weak spots" more likely to fail under stress—which will be especially concerning for load-bearing implants such as for bone or cartilage regeneration.

patentable [23]. As far as Kritikos [23]; is concerned, in his research, the European Legislation will have to face the following questions:

- sufficiency of the law
- the number of involved individuals
- who would be coauthors of a work
- patentable new biological matter
- line between the living and the nonliving in biotechnology
- legal method of bioprinting

Many of the metal materials that are generally used for permanent implants have a high elastic modulus, which often leads to an elastic mismatch between the implant

Table 5.3 New risks inherent to bioprinting organ? [31].

Technology	Risk linked to purpose of printing parts of body
3D bioprinting	Unlike most structures implanted in the body (stents, pacemakers, cochlear implants, artificial hips, or knees), bioprinted engineered tissue initiates an ongoing interaction with the recipient's body, and variations may not be controllable. This has consequences for accurate risk–benefit analysis and for the results of clinical trials.
	Quality control limitations may give rise to additional risks for bioprinting due to the variability of the tissues and products that are printed.
	The problem of quality control for printed organs: It may be possible to test the function of some organs, such as the heart, prior to implantation. However, other organs, such as a kidney, play such complex roles within the body that their function cannot be fully assessed in the lab.
	Even if efficacy of a transplanted artificial organ is demonstrated for one human, the results may not be generalizable to others in the population. Each individual organ is a stand-alone, personalized treatment, a complex machine with thousands of working parts.
	An organ, e.g., kidney, generated from a patient's own cells may replicate the genetic disposition of that individual which caused the original organ to fail—resulting in a recurring problem. These consequences may not become apparent for several years and so may not be determinable in a short-term safety trial.
	Even biologically inert materials can have unexpected, possibly unforeseeable, consequences.

and the bone. Printed biodegradable scaffolds are generally fabricated from natural polymers with good biocompatibility but poor mechanical properties, such as collagen, sodium alginate, and other hydrogels. In addition, international standards for choosing medical materials for 3D printing have not been developed; thus, only synthetic evaluations can be made based on structure, function, clinical effects, and other aspects, rather than evaluations based on reliable indicators and sufficient experimental evidence [32].

Computer-aided 3D printing approaches to the industrial production of customized 3D functional living constructs for restoration of tissue and organ function face significant regulatory challenges. Existing EU and US regulatory frameworks do not account for the differences between 3D printing and conventional manufacturing methods or the ability to create individual customized products using mechanized rather than craft approaches. Already subject to extensive regulatory control, issues related to control of the computer-aided design to manufacture process and the associated software system chain, present additional scientific and regulatory challenges for manufacturers of these complex 3D-bioprinted advanced combination products [33].

The rules governing the placement of human medicines on the market in the EU and the United States are broadly divided under public health and core pharmaceutical and medical device legislation. Pharmaceuticals, biologics, and medical devices are subject to different regulatory requirements that govern premarket applications, manufacturing practices, and postmarket reporting of adverse events. In the United States, the Code of Federal Regulations (Title 21 CFR), based on the Federal Food, Drug, and Cosmetic Act (FD&C Act) and the Public Health Service Act (PHS Act), establishes the legal framework within which the US FDA regulates the distribution and sale of medical products. These legal instruments provide the precise product definition and legal basis for classification of products as drugs, biologics, medical devices, or combination products. Each of the product types is regulated by a different office within the FDA, either the Center for Drug Evaluation and Research (CDER), the Center for Biologics Evaluation and Research (CBER), or the Center for Devices and Radiological Health (CDRH). In the EU, a relevant product can only be regulated as either a medicinal product (whether drug or biologic) or a medical device, as classified by the applicable and legally separate sector-specific legislation that differ markedly in terms of procedures to be followed to place the product on the EU market [33].

Lastly, regarding data protection of the patient, the basic question has to do with patient privacy consent for the 3D printing of their organs, the principles of the procedure, what happens after the surgery, etc.

EU regulations for medical 3D printing products

The new Medical Devices Regulation (2017/745/European Union (EU)) (MDR) and the *In Vitro* Diagnostic Medical Devices Regulation (2017/746/EU) (IVDR) bring EU legislation into line with technical advances, changes in medical science, and progress in law making. The new Regulations create a robust, transparent, and sustainable regulatory framework, recognized internationally, that improves clinical safety and creates fair market access for manufacturers. In contrast to Directives, Regulations do not need to be transposed into national law. The MDR and the IVDR will therefore reduce the risks of discrepancies in interpretation across the EU market.[c] The new legislation contains

- Clinical evaluation;
- Risk management;
- Quality Management System (QMS);
- Postmarket surveillance;
- Technical documentation and other reports; and
- Liability for defective devices.

Specifically, the Regulation (EU) 2017/745 of the European Parliament and of the Council of 5 April 2017 on medical devices, amending Directive 2001/83/EC,

---

[c] https://ec.europa.eu/growth/sectors/medical-devices_en.

Regulation (EC) No 178/2002 and Regulation (EC) No 1223/2009 and repealing Council Directives 90/385/EEC and 93/42/EEC and more specifically paragraphs 2,10,20,21 [23]:

- **Paragraph 2:** *"This Regulation aims to ensure the smooth functioning of the internal market as regards medical devices, taking as a base a high level of protection of health for patients and users, and taking into account the small- and medium-sized enterprises that are active in this sector. At the same time, this Regulation sets high standards of quality and safety for medical devices in order to meet common safety concerns as regards such products. Both objectives are being pursued simultaneously and are inseparably linked whilst one not being secondary to the other. As regards Article 114 of the Treaty on the Functioning of the European Union (TFEU), this Regulation harmonises the rules for the placing on the market and putting into service of medical devices and their accessories on the Union market thus allowing them to benefit from the principle of free movement of goods."*

- **Paragraph 10**: *"Products which combine a medicinal product or substance and a medical device are regulated either under this Regulation or under Directive 2001/83/EC of the European Parliament and of the Council. (3) The two legislative acts should ensure appropriate interaction in terms of consultations during pre-market assessment, and of exchange of information in the context of vigilance activities involving such combination products. For medicinal products that integrate a medical device part, compliance with the general safety and performance requirements laid down in this Regulation for the device part should be adequately assessed in the context of the marketing authorisation for such medicinal products. Directive 2001/83/EC should therefore be amended"*.

- **Paragraph 20:** *"The definitions in this Regulation, regarding devices themselves, the making available of devices, economic operators, users and specific processes, the conformity assessment, clinical investigations and clinical evaluations, post-market surveillance, vigilance and market surveillance, standards and other technical specifications, should be aligned with well-established practice in the field at Union and international level in order to enhance legal certainty. (21) It should be made clear that it is essential that devices offered to persons in the Union by means of information society services within the meaning of Directive (EU) 2015/1535 of the European Parliament and of the Council (1) and devices used in the context of a commercial activity to provide a diagnostic or therapeutic service to persons within the Union comply with the requirements of this Regulation, where the product in question is placed on the market or the service is provided in the Union"*.

- **Paragraph 21:** *"It should be made clear that it is essential that devices offered to persons in the Union by means of information society services within the meaning of Directive (EU) 2015/1535 of the European Parliament and of the Council (1) and devices used in the context of a commercial activity to provide a diagnostic or therapeutic service to persons within the Union comply with the* *requirements of this Regulation, where the product in question is placed on the market or the service is provided in the Union."*

Conclusions

The Regulation (EU) 2017/745 assures improvement of the quality, safety and reliability of medical devices, transparency of information for consumers, and enhancement of vigilance and market surveillance. 3D bioprinting has proven to be a great success in major applications in pharmaceutics, medicine, and dentistry. More specifically, great progress has been made in the field of in dental and orthodontic treatments, tissue engineering, drug development, and orthopedic implants, just to name a few of the multiple applications of 3D printing.

Medical biomaterials used in 3D printing consist of metals, polymers, and ceramics, with multiple materials usually being integrated in order to achieve complex functions in the printed components. Although 3D printing has already been involved in clinical applications, 3D printing technology is still limited in terms of materials and in the construction of Extracellular matrix (ECM) *in vitro* [32]. Regarding these limitations, [23] argues that they primarily have to do with: law sufficient IP, the number of involved individuals, who would be coauthors of a work, patentable new biological matter line between the living and the nonliving in biotechnology and legal method of bioprinting.

Overall, we can see that we are clearly at a stage where we are starting to realize the full potential of 3D printing, as well as the challenges involved in realizing that potential. Chief among them are the issues of quality and safety, as no matter what the potential advantage of 3D printing is, these are principles that cannot be sacrificed [34].

References

[1] Prasad L, Smyth H. 3D Printing technologies for drug delivery: a review. Drug Dev Ind Pharm 2015;42:1019−31.

[2] Kizawa H, Nagao E, Shimamura M, Zhang G, Torii H. Scaffold-free 3D bioprinted human liver tissue stably maintains metabolic functions useful for drug discovery. Biochem Biophys Rep 2017;10:186−91.

[3] Munoz-Abraham A, Rodriguez-Davalos M, Bertacco A, Wengerter B, Geibel J, Mulligan D. 3D printing of organs for transplantation: where are we and where are we heading? Curr Transplant Rep 2016;3:93−9.

[4] Ferris C, Gilmore K, Beirne S, McCallum D, Wallace G, in het Panhuis M. Bioink for on-demand printing of living cells. Biomater Sci 2013;1:224−30.

[5] Spritamcom Spritam (2017), Available at: https://www.spritam.com.

[6] Shende P, Agrawal S. Integration of 3D printing with dosage forms: a new perspective for modern healthcare. Biomed Pharmacother 2018;107:146−54.

[7] Available at: Basiliere P. Gartner Predicts 2016: 3D printing Disrupts healthcare and manufacturing — Pete Basiliere. 2017. https://blogs.gartner.com/pete-basiliere/2015/12/02/gartner-predicts-2016-3Dprinting- disrupts-healthcare-and-manufacturing/.

[8] Sheikh A, Chepelev L, Christensen AM, Mitsouras D, Schwarz BA, Rybicki FJ. Beginning and developing a radiology-based in-hospital 3D printing lab. In: Rybicki F, Grant G, editors. 3D printing in medicine; 2017.

[9] Malik HH, Darwood ARJ, Shaunak S, Kulatilake P, El-Hilly AA, Mulki O, Baskaradas A. Three-dimensional printing in surgery: a review of current surgical applications. J Surg Res 2015;199(2):512—22.

[10] Yang L, Grottkau B, He Z, Ye CL. Three dimensional printing technology and materials for treatment of elbow fractures. Int Orthop 2017;41(11):2381—7.

[11] Atalay HA, Canat HL, Ülker V, Alkan İ, Özkuvanci Ü, Altunrende F. Impact of personalized three-dimensional (3D)printed pelvicalyceal system models on patient information in percutaneous nephrolithotripsy surgery: a pilot study. Int Braz J Urol 2017;43(3): 470—5.

[12] Li K, Kui C, Lee E, Ho C, Wong S, Wu W, Wong W, Voll J, Li G, Liu T, Yan B, Chan J, Tse G, Keenan I. The role of 3D printing in anatomy education and surgical training: a narrative review. MedEdPublish 2017;6(2):31.

[13] Sodian R, Weber S, Markert M, Loeff M, Tim Lueth T, Weis FC, Daebritz S, Malec E, Schmitz C, Reichart B. Pediatric cardiac transplantation: three-dimensional printing of anatomic models for surgical planning of heart transplantation in patients with univentricular heart. J Thorac Cardiovasc Surg 2008;136(4):1098—9.

[14] Zheng Y, Yu D, Zhao J, Wu Y, Zheng B. 3D printout models vs. 3D-rendered images: which is better for preoperative planning? J Surg Educ 2016;73(3):518—23.

[15] Auricchio F, Marconi S. 3D printing: clinical applications in orthopaedics and traumatology. EFORT Open Rev 2016;1(5):121—7.

[16] Parthasarathy J. 3D modeling, custom implants and its future perspectives in craniofacial surgery. Ann Maxillofac Surg 2014;4(1):9—18.

[17] Hong C. Application of 3D printing in orthopedics: status quo and opportunities in China. Ann Transl Med 2015;3(S1):S12.

[18] Leng S, McGee K, Morris J, Alexander A, Kuhlmann J, Vrieze T, McCollough CH, Matsumoto J. Anatomic modeling using 3D printing: quality assurance and optimization. 3D Print Med 2017;3—6.

[19] Kanters D, deVries A, Boon H, Urbach J, Becht A, Kooistra H-A. Quality assurance in medical 3D-printing. In: Lhotska L, et al., editors. World congress on medical physics and biomedical engineering 2018,IFMBE Proceedings 68/1; 2018. https://doi.org/10.1007/978-981-10-9035-6_125.

[20] Sampat N, Kulkarni R, Sase N, Joshi N, Vora P, Bhattacharya A, Lakhani J, Bhowmik S. Once daily baclofen sustained release or gastro-retentive system are acceptable alternatives to thrice daily baclofen immediate release at same daily dosage in patients. Neurol India 2009;57:295—9.

[21] Scoutaris N, Ross SA, Douroumis D. 3D printed "starmix" drug loaded dosage forms for paediatric applications. Pharm Res 2018;35:34.

[22] Palekar S, Nukala PK, Mishra SM, Kipping T, Patel K. Application of 3D printing technology and quality by design approach for development of age-appropriate pediatric formulation of baclofen. Int J Pharm 2019;556:106—16.

[23] Kritikos M. 3D bioprinting for medical and enhancement purposes: legal and ethical aspects. european parliamentary research service (EPRS). In-Depth analysis,scientific

foresight unit (STOA), PE 614.571, European Parliament, July 2018, European Union. 2018.

[24] Lopez FL, Ernest TB, Tuleu C, Gul MO. Formulation approaches to pediatric oral drug delivery: benefits and limitations of current platforms. Exp Opin Drug Deliv 2015;12: 1727−40.

[25] Martina M, Hutmacher DW. Biodegradable polymers applied in tissue engineering research: a review. Polym Int 2007;56(2):145−57.

[26] Ratner BD, Bryant SJ. Biomaterials: where we have been and where we are going. Annu Rev Biomed Eng 2004;6:41−75.

[27] Hyun I. The bioethics of stem cell research and therapy. J Clin Investig 2010;120:71−5.

[28] Nair K, Gandhi M, Khalil S, Yan KC, Marcolongo M, Barbee K, et al. Characterization of cell viability during bioprinting processes. Biotechnol J 2009;4(8):1168−77.

[29] Hilleman MR. Discovery of simian virus 40 (SV40) and its relationship to poliomyelitis virus vaccines. Dev Biol Stand 1998;94:183−90.

[30] Atala A, Bauer SB, Soker S, Yoo JJ, Retik AB. Tissue-engineered autologous bladders for patients needing cystoplasty. Lancet 2006;367(9518):1241−6.

[31] Gilbert F, O'Connell CD, Mladenovska T, Dodds S. Print me an organ? ethical and regulatory issues emerging from 3D bioprinting in medicine. Sprieger 2015.

[32] Yan, Dong H, Su J, Han J, Song B, Wei Q, Shi Y. A review of 3D printing technology for medical applications. Engineering 2018;4(5):729−42. https://doi.org/10.1016/j.eng. 2018.07.021.

[33] Hourd P, Medcalf N, Segal J, Williams D. A 3D-bioprinting exemplar of the consequences of the regulatory requirements on customized processes. Regen Med 2015; 10(7):863−83.

[34] Available at: United States Government Accountability Office. 3D printing: opportunities, challenges, and policy implications of additive manufacturing. 2015. http://www.gao.gov/assets/680/670960.pdf.

Economics in 3D printing

Nikitas Nikitakos[1], Ioannis Dagkinis, PhD[2], Dimitrios Papachristos, PhD[3], Georgios Georgantis, MD, PhD[4], Evanthia Kostidi, PhD[2]

[1]*Professor, Department of Shipping Trade & Transport, University of the Aegean, Chios, Greece;* [2]*Department of Shipping Trade & Transport, University of the Aegean, Chios, Greece;* [3]*University of West Attica, Greece;* [4]*Academic Fellow, Aristotle University of Thessaloniki, Thessaloniki, Greece*

Introduction

Additive manufacturing (AM), or 3D printing, as it is more commonly known, is already been augmented in various industries like automotive, aircraft, medical industry, just to name a few. The American Society for Testing and Materials (ASTM) groups them in seven different categories.

As far as Grand View Research is concerned the 3D printing market is divided into three categories: raw materials, application, and region. The 3D printing industry has one of the highest projections for economic growth. McKinsey estimates that 3D printing market could reach $180–490 billion by 2025. The health market industry which includes the medical sector and the dental laboratories has a great impact on the 3D printing market growth.

Additive manufacturing (3D printing) technology

AM, although it has been around for more than 30 years, is commonly known to the general public as 3D printing. It is based upon the principle of the construction in layers by adding material, differentiating the process from molding, or removing material, for example, in the lathe. It has been already implemented in various sectors (industrial products, consumer products, automotive, aerospace, medicine, etc.).

Synonyms are additive fabrication, additive processes, additive techniques, additive layer manufacturing, layer manufacturing, and freeform fabrication.

AM is the official industry standard term (ASTM F2792) for all applications of the technology. It is defined as the process of joining materials to make objects from 3D model data, usually layer upon layer, as opposed to subtractive manufacturing methodologies.

3D Printing: Applications in Medicine and Surgery. https://doi.org/10.1016/B978-0-323-66164-5.00006-4

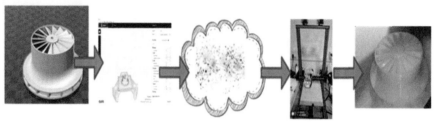

FIGURE 6.1

From the 3D model to the actual printed part.[1].

Source: Kostidi and Nikitakos (2018).

The start of process is a digital file of the item that can be created using a CAD tool, or digitized if already existing (by a scanner or tomography). Having the design of a product is the first step for printing it (making it additively), that can be made anywhere in the world (providing a suitable machine and the raw material). Fig. 6.1 shows the process of building the part from the 3D digital model.

Under the umbrella of AM there are many processes. ASTM groups them in seven types (Fig. 6.2):

1) **Binder jetting**—AM process where a liquid bonding agent is deposited to join powdered materials together.
2) **Direct energy deposition (direct manufacturing)**—AM process where thermal energy fuses or melts materials together as they are added.
3) **Material extrusion (fused deposition modeling)**—AM process that allows for depositing material via a nozzle.
4) **Material jetting**—AM process where droplets of material are deposited.
5) **Powder bed fusion (laser sintering)**—AM process where thermal energy fuses or melts material from a powder bed.
6) **Sheet welding (e-beam welding, laminated object manufacturing)**—AM process where sheets of materials are bonded together.

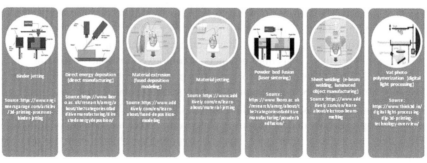

FIGURE 6.2

The seven processes of additive manufacturing by ASTM.

7) Vat photo-polymerization (digital light processing)—AM process where liquid photopolymer in vat is cured by light.

In some processes the material is squirted, squeezed, or sprayed and in others fused, bound, or glued. The power source is thermal, high-powered laser beam, electron beam, ultraviolet laser, or photo curing.

The raw materials for the process are polymers, metals, ceramics, composites, and biological materials. The starting materials could be liquid, filament/paste, powder, or solid sheet. Currently, the most common metallic materials are steels (tool steel and stainless), pure titanium and titanium alloys, aluminum casting alloys, nickel-based super alloys, cobalt-chromium alloys, gold, and silver [2].

It is possible to realize high shape complexity without increasing the production costs (contrary to traditional technology). Freedom of design impacts the weight of the object that can be made lighter. Reduction of weight has an impact on lifecycle cost, material cost, and energy consumption in the production phase.

Additive technology has various advantages and disadvantages. Some of these have been identified by Lindemann et al. (2012) and are listed below.

Advantages:

- More flexible development
- Freedom of design and construction
- Less assembly
- No production tool necessary
- Less spare parts in stock
- Less complexity in business because less parts to manage
- Less time to market for products
- Faster deployment of changes

Disadvantages:

- High machine and material costs
- Quality of parts is in need of improvement
- Rework is often necessary (support structures)
- Building time depends on the height of the part in the building chamber

The market structure of additive manufacturing (3D printing) industry

Markets for AM could hence be characterized by four patterns [3]:

- Small production output, as typical for prototyping applications but also many industrial components or especially spare parts for older product families still in use.
- High product complexity, as typical for lightweight constructions in the aerospace or performance car industries (AM allows the manufacture of mash

structures that provide the same performance effect by largely reduced material usage), but also for product designs where current production technologies like molding or milling cannot provide complicated internal structures such as cooling chambers.

- High demand for product customization tailored to individual customers' needs, as typical for many medical or dental applications (implants, prostheses) but also consumer markets like jewelry or sport performance products.
- Spatially remote demand for products, for example, the decentralized production of replacement parts in the mining industry or on exploitation platforms of the oil industry.

As far as Grand View Research (Grand View Research, 2014), the 3D printing market is divided into three categories (Fig. 6.3):

- Raw materials
- Application
- Region

To begin with raw materials, Grand View Research (Grand View Research, 2014) shows 36.9% use of polymers, 33.9% ceramic goods, and 22.6% metals (Fig. 6.4).

As for industries, the highest percentage of growth is shown by the automotive industry with 40.5%, then the aerospace with 23.3%. The medical sector and the dental laboratories gather 18.2% (Grand View Research, 2014) (Fig. 6.5).

Examining regions, North America comes first with 42.2%, then Europe with 36.5% and Asia Pacific with 11.5%. The economy ministry of Japan, which is the

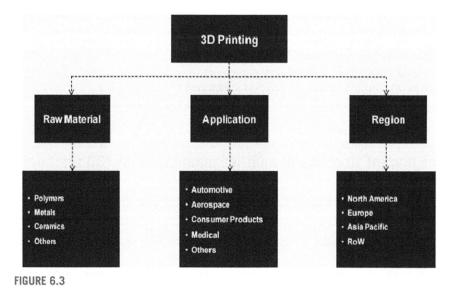

FIGURE 6.3

3D printing market segmentation.

Source: Grand View Research (2014).

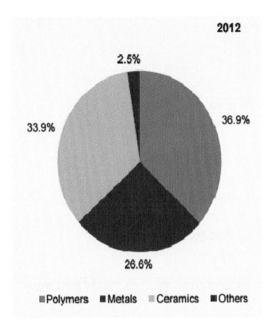

FIGURE 6.4

3D printing market raw materials segmentation.

Source: Grand View Research (2014).

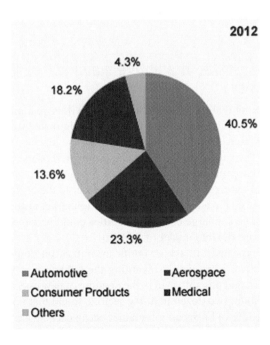

FIGURE 6.5

3D printing market by application segmentation.

Source: Grand View Research (2014).

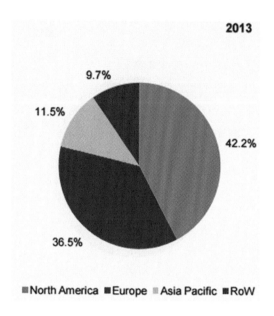

2013

9.7%

11.5%

42.2%

36.5%

■North America ■Europe ■Asia Pacific ■RoW

FIGURE 6.6

3D printing market by region segmentation.

Source: Grand View Research (2014).

largest market of Asia, is aiming to include USD 44 million in the budget by the use of the new technology (Grand View Research, 2014) (Fig. 6.6).

The economic growth of additive manufacturing (3D printing) industry

Market surveys predict that the introduction of AM will have a major impact on industries and manufacturing [3]. The new technology eliminated stages of production (e.g., assembly) and thus simplified production line. The place of production moves closer to demand. The sale is made before the production of the product, upsetting the known production process.

The production facilities can now be located closer to the customer in Europe or North America, resulting in a more direct response to market needs [4]. The concept of constructing products in large complex facilities could become obsolete as companies adopt the more flexible model of AM [5].

3D printing is expected to have a significant impact on domestic and international freight operators, in particular regarding the reduction of the importance of some transport paths, and possibly lead to the opening of new ones. A recent analysis [6] for Strategy&, about two dozen industry sectors, found that up to 41% of the air cargo business and 37% of businesses container ocean carriers are at risk because of 3D printing.

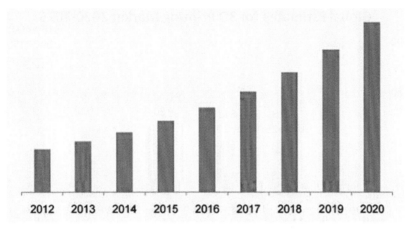

FIGURE 6.7

Global 3D Printing market revenue (USD Million), 2012–2020.

Source: Grand View Research (2014).

Ye et al. [7], based on a model, conclude that in the next 2 decades, 3D printing is not likely to pose a threat, on the concept of significant production capacity, or reduce the transport flow, in terms of global container traffic. As the GDP of the world's population is not likely to decline over the next 50 years, world trade will probably continue to cause high demand for transport.

"The global market for 3D printing was estimated to be USD 2183 million in 2012, and is expected to reach USD 8675.7 million by 2020, growing at a CAGR of 18.9% from 2013 to 2020" (Grand View Research, 2014) (Fig. 6.7).

According to Wohlers Report 2018: "In 2017, the AM industry, consisting of all AM products and services worldwide, grew 21% to $7.336 billion. The growth in 2017 compares to 17.4% growth in 2016 when the industry reached $6.063 billion and 25.9% growth in 2015" (Wohlers Report, 2018).

The ARK Invest (2016) summarizes in a chart the growth projections from reputable firms. As it can be seen in Fig. 6.8, McKinsey estimates that 3D printing market could reach $180–490 billion by 2025. The 3D printing industry has one of the highest projections for economic growth.

3D printing in health market

As already shown in the previous paragraphs, the health market industry which includes the medical sector and the dental laboratories has a great impact on the 3D printing market growth.

The healthcare 3D printing market, that will be more thoroughly examined in the following chapters by specialty applications, is divided into three categories (Fig. 6.9):

• Medical

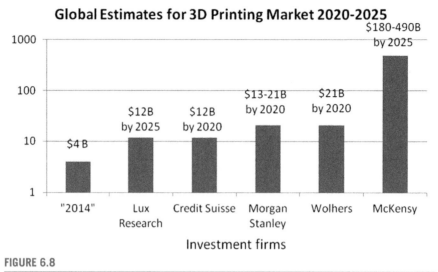

FIGURE 6.8

Global estimates for 3D printing market, 2020—25.

Source: ARK Invest (2016).

- Dental
- Biosensors

Medical applications are mainly grouped into three categories:

- Pharmaceutical
- Prosthetics and Implants
- Tissue and Organ Generation

"The global healthcare 3D printing market size was valued at USD 578.0 million in 2017 and is anticipated to grow at a significant CAGR over the forecast period. Growing demand for customized 3D printed devices and implants should drive healthcare 3D printing market size over the forecast period." As depicted from Global Market Insights, the highest percentage of 3D printing in health industry by region comes from Europe and North America (Fig. 6.10) [8].

Conclusion—further research

Among the benefits of AM is the flexible production of customized products, in small batches. The direct transformation of the three-dimensional data stored in a file, simply by supplying the raw materials to the machine and the production of natural objects, obviating the need for the assembly step can be applied to the manufacture of products near the place where they are needed.

It has already an increased presence in various industries like automotive, aircraft, medical industry, among others. The ASTM groups them in seven different

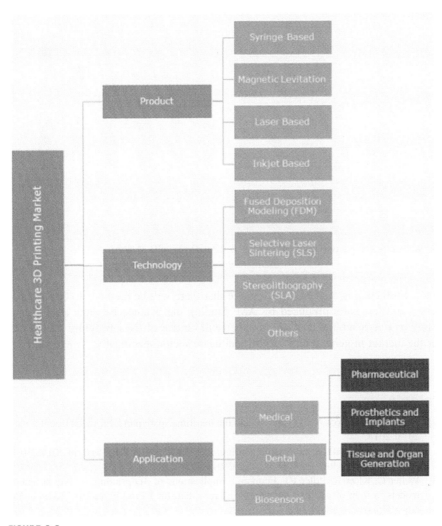

FIGURE 6.9

Industry segmentation in Global healthcare 3D printing.

Source: Healthcare 3D printing market global market Insights 2018.

categories. Grand View Research divides the 3D printing market into three categories: raw materials, application, and region. The 3D printing industry has one of the highest projections for economic growth. The health market industry which includes the medical sector and the dental laboratories has a great impact on the 3D printing market growth.

The main skepticism for the products made by AM is the quality of the part, and the cost of the printing machines/material and consequently the price of the so made

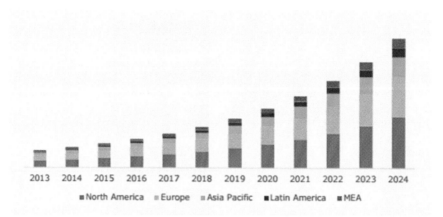

FIGURE 6.10

Global healthcare 3D printing market size, 2013—2024 (USD Million).

Source: Healthcare 3D printing market global market Insights 2018.

items. Forthcoming standards will assure that there will be methods to ensure processes and test parts produced by AM. Finding the balance between quality and safety on one hand and cost on the other will be one of the key future challenges for the market in general and for the healthcare sector specifically.

References

[1] Kostidi E, Nikitakos N. 3D Printing and the maritime spare parts. In: ELINT conference 2018; 2018.

[2] Frazier WE. Metal additive manufacturing: a review. J Mater Eng Perform 2014;23(6): 1917—28. https://doi.org/10.1007/s11665-014-0958-z.

[3] Weller C, Kleer R, Piller FT. Economic implications of 3D printing: market structure models in light of additive manufacturing revisited. Int J Prod Econ 2015;164:43—56. https://doi.org/10.1016/j.ijpe.2015.02.020.

[4] Manners-Bell J, Lyon K. The implications of 3D printing for the global logistics industry. Transp Intell 2012;1—5.

[5] Cottrill K. Transforming the future of supply chains through disruptive innovation. MIT Center for Transportation and Logistics; 2011. Working Paper, Spring. Retrieved from: http://www.misi.edu.my/student/spv1/assets/Disruptive_Innovations4_1.pdf.

[6] Tipping A, Schmahl A, Duiven F. 2015 commercial transportation trends. 2015. Retrieved 12 June 2016, from: http://www.strategyand.pwc.com/perspectives/2015-commercial-transportation-trends.

[7] Ye M, Tavasszy LA, Van Duin JHR, Wiegmans B, Halim RA, TU Delft: Technology, Policy and Management: Transport and Logistics, TU Delft, Delft University of Technology. The impact of 3D printing on the world container transport. March 12, 2015. Retrieved from: http://resolver.tudelft.nl/uuid:f16ee590-5804-4beb-b72c-a32346d0f175.

[8] Healthcare 3D printing market global market insights; 2018.

Further reading

[1] ASTM 2013. AM_Standards_Development_Plan_v2.docx (n.d.). Retrieved from: http://www.astm.org/COMMIT/AM_Standars_Development_Plan_v2.docx.

[2] https://wohlersassociates.com/press74.html.

[3] 3D printing market analysis and segment forecasts to 2020 Grand View research 2018.

Three-dimensional (3D) printing and liver transplantation

Ioannis A. Ziogas, MD [1,4], Nizar N. Zein, MD [2,5,6], Cristiano Quintini, MD [3,7], Charles M. Miller, MD [3,8], Georgios Tsoulfas, MD, PhD [9]

[1]*First Department of Surgery, Aristotle University of Thessaloniki, Thessaloniki, Greece;* [2]*Department of Gastroenterology and Hepatology, Digestive Disease Institute, Cleveland Clinic, Cleveland, OH, United States;* [3]*Department of Hepato-Pancreato-Biliary and Transplant Surgery, Digestive Disease Institute, Cleveland Clinic, Cleveland, OH, United States;* [4]*Postdoctoral Research Fellow, Division of Hepatobiliary Surgery and Liver Transplantation, Section of Surgical Sciences, Vanderbilt University Medical Center, Nashville, TN, United States;* [5]*Director, Mikati Liver Center, Digestive Disease and Surgery Institute, The Cleveland Clinic, Cleveland, OH, United States;* [6]*Chair, Global Patient Services, The Cleveland Clinic, Cleveland, OH, United States;* [7]*Director, Associate Professor of Surgery, Cleveland Clinic Lerner College of Medicine, Liver Tranpslantation, General Surgery, Cleveland Clinic, Cleveland, OH, United States;* [8]*Enterprise Director of Transplantation, Transplantation Center, Digestive Disease and Surgery Institute, Cleveland, OH, United States;* [9]*Associate Professor, Department of Surgery, Aristotle University of Thessaloniki, Thessaloniki, Greece*

Introduction

Anatomical knowledge is a cornerstone and an essential part for the performance of successful surgical and invasive procedures. A number of studies suggested a relation between the volume of surgeries performed and the rate of complications, including mortality. This association has been attributed, at least in part, to the incomplete characterization of anatomical structures in a way to account for individual variations [1,2]. Even from the medical-legal perspective, a substantial number of claims have directly attributed to anatomical errors leading to an unintended "damage" of nearby structures [3]. In an effort to optimize outcomes, the surgeon used a wide range of preoperative planning techniques in order to improve efficiency, diminish operative time, and ultimately reduce the incidence of surgical complications. The widespread use of imaging for preoperative planning of high-risk surgical procedures provided accuracy and improved knowledge of anatomical variations [4−6]. Additional approaches beyond standard imaging were more recently introduced to assist in surgical planning and for risk analysis of individual cases, including computer-assisted three-dimensional (3D) imaging and the use of surgical models. These techniques provided enhanced intraoperative orientation. 3D printing has recently been applied as an advanced tool with properties and potential advantages of both 3D imaging and physical surgical models where individual patient's imaging is used to replicate the authentic anatomy of the person to undergo surgery.

3D printing, also known as rapid prototyping or additive manufacturing, involves the implementation of various techniques in order to "translate" a computer-generated image into a 3D solid object by printing consecutive thin layers of a specific type of material [7]. 3D printing became widely available after the expiration of patents in 2009 and the subsequent drop in printer prices [8]. Converting the two-dimensional (2D) image into 3D is of paramount importance in medicine and particularly in surgical specialties, and consequently, the medical industry could not help but embrace this opportunity. Besides, the evolution of surgery over the past century has been closely associated with various technological advancements. Now, 3D printed anatomic models have already started to make valuable inroads into surgical planning and execution.

It is accepted that 3D imaging tools are superior to 2D in terms of orienting anatomical structures that help the surgeon create a solid preoperative plan. However, studying 3D images on a 2D screen imposes its limitations. The 2D screen entails the difficulty of accurately estimating the depth of the image, and hence the 3D printed object allows for the precise resemblance of the cutting planes and the intraoperative setting with a significant increase in spatial perception. In addition, surgeons can manipulate the organ and orient themselves, which makes it easier to identify critical anatomical landmarks and the most comfortable physical position in the operating room (OR), as well as understand how to achieve optimal exposure intraoperatively.

So far, the surgical fields witnessing most of the applications of 3D printing are oral and maxillofacial surgery and orthopedic surgery [9], neurosurgery [10], and cardiac surgery [11]. Transplantation surgery, and liver transplantation, in particular, is a novel field of medicine that rapidly evolved technically after overcoming the many immunological hurdles inherent in transplantation. Arguably, solid organ transplantation, including liver transplantation, is a complex, multistep process that requires impeccable surgery from start to finish. Accordingly, greater preoperative preparation, including an anatomical understanding of the individual patient, will likely improve outcomes and decreases the likelihood for surgical complications.

Today, liver transplantation has become an everyday practice, primarily due to the reduction in contraindications and the expansion of transplantation criteria. Nevertheless, it is apparent that the largest challenge today in liver transplantation is the existing discrepancy between the shortage of donor organs and the ever-growing number of patients awaiting a graft. The new era of partial liver grafting, especially with living donor segments and lobes, has become a fertile ground for the development and application of 3D printing. Using 3D printed models has a special benefit for preoperative planning, intraoperative execution, and medical education.

3D printing technologies

3D printing is a term used to describe a series of technologies that are used to build functional parts for many different uses. The common feature among all of these technologies is that the part is built by adding horizontal layers of material sequentially in the vertical direction. It is similar in principle to building a part out of Lego blocks—typically the base layer is built, and additional blocks are added piece by piece in order to achieve the final shape. In both the example of the Lego block as well as every 3D printing technology, the build method is additive in nature. This may be contrasted with more traditional methods of manufacturing, such as machining (material is sequentially removed from a starting shape) or molding (a liquid material is forced into a mold and then cooled into a solid), in order to achieve the desired geometry.

Historically, 3D printing referred to one of several specific technologies. General terms to describe these technologies include solid freeform fabrication, rapid prototyping, and additive manufacturing. Of these, additive manufacturing best describes the term 3D printing as it is readily understood by the public.

3D printing got its start with Charles Hull, who invented the Stereolithography Apparatus, or "SLA." He patented this technology in 1986 (Patent #US4575330); this patent was the technological basis for the company 3D Systems, which released the first commercially available SLA machine in 1988. In the following years, additional technologies were introduced, including Fused Deposition Modeling ("FDM") in 1991 (Stratasys, Edina, Minnesota, United States), Selective Laser Sintering ("SLS") in 1992 (3D Systems, Rock Hill, South Carolina, United States), and PBP (3D Systems) in 1996. In more recent years, the Polyjet (Stratasys) machines and several variations of metal laser sintering, including Direct Metal Laser Sintering ("DMLS") (3D Systems; EOS, EOS GmbH, Krailling, Germany) were introduced. Each of these technologies has unique characteristics, and therefore potentially unique applications in medicine.

There are several advantages inherent in 3D printing technologies in comparison with traditional manufacturing methods. Perhaps the most important advantage of 3D printing is that virtually any shape, no matter the complexity, can be built. This feature is highly advantageous for medical applications given the complexity of anatomical structures of individual organs such as the human liver. Other key advantages of 3D printing technologies are the speed of fabrication and simplicity of the process. All 3D printing technologies rely on the operator supplying a digital file called an STL file (derived from the word "stereolithography"). The STL file contains coordinates that define triangles that, in turn, represent the geometry of the part to be built. Design engineers would typically use the Computer-Aided Design (CAD) software package they are using to design the prototype to generate an STL file for 3D printing of that prototype.

Medical education and training

Interpretation of 3D anatomical information has always been an integral part of medical education and is the backbone of understanding disease processes and invasive interventions such as surgery. 3D printing has the potential to be highly innovative and effective new modality in a number of disciplines associated with educations and training (Fig. 7.1).

With the rapid advancement of medical imaging, knowledge of human anatomy, and the 3D relationship of its components has become an even more important element of training. Classical anatomical education utilized a combination of teaching modalities including cadaveric dissection (considered the benchmark of anatomy classes in most medical schools), which has several advantages not offered by alternative methods such as 2D visual representation [12]. Cadaveric dissection offers the means for learning anatomical 3D spatial relationship, allows understanding of anatomical variability among individuals, and involves tactile manipulation of structures. However, the availability of cadavers is increasingly more limited, while ethical justification surrounding their use has been questioned [13].

Besides cadaveric-based training, medical institutions have relied heavily on the 2D visual representation of complex 3D human anatomy, a method that has been an association with a detrimental increase in cognitive load and subsequently less retention of information [14]. The recognition of these shortcomings led to the

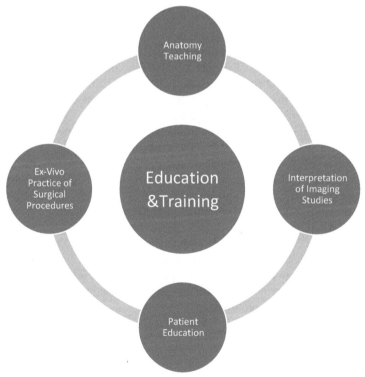

FIGURE 7.1

The four distinct areas of Education and Medical Training, where patient-specific 3D printing is likely beneficial.

development of computer-assisted 3D anatomical models, which is considered more enjoyable and stimulating to students than tradition 2D visual illustrations [15,16]. These newer computer-assisted techniques were intended to overcome some of the difficulties of understanding the 3D nature of human anatomy but have also been associated with similarly high and detrimental cognitive overload in students with limited innate spatial capabilities [17].

3D printing of human anatomical components, while untested broadly in classrooms, may provide an alternative teaching tool with combined advantages of computer-assisted 3D representation (understand 3D spatial relationships) even for students with limited innate spatial capacities and of cadaveric-based learning including tactile manipulation and appreciation of individual anatomical variability among persons. 3D printed anatomical models are derived from individual patient imaging studies and are identical copies to the actual anatomical part of the patient used for the creation of these models. 3D printing allows for creativity in the selection of the materials used for printing including the use of transparent materials for solid organ, allowing for an understanding of the complex vascular and nonvascular structures within the specific organ studied. The use of colored materials where newer 3D printers can simultaneously incorporate multiple colors will likely enhance learning above and beyond cadaveric-based lessons where structures are distorted and of uniform color. Finally, a medical school may potentially have a collection of 3D printed model derived from patients with anatomical variations, a task that is impossible to achieve with cadavers.

Another aspect of medical education in which 3D printing may enrich is the interpretation of imaging studies often incorporated in the training of Radiology, Surgical, and Medical residents. The integration of interactive 3D imaging into undergraduate radiology education have shown to effectively improve radiological reasoning, visual-spatial ability, diagnostic skills, and confidence [18]. We propose that the availability of a 3D printed physical model derived from a patient-specific imaging study can significantly enhance visual/spatial appreciation of anatomy with complex spatial relationship and improve the ability of interpretation. This possibility was tested in students of veterinary medicine using 3D printed physical models as a novel teaching tool compared to 2D and 3D imaging of equine foot [19]. Investigators demonstrated that the physical models hold a significant advantage over alternative learning methods (2D and 3D imaging) in understanding complex anatomical architecture [19]. Incorporating imaging with 3D physical models may well provide a great and novel teaching tool to augment the talent of students in visually converting 2D/3D image findings into a realistic 3D structure consistent with human anatomy.

The Cleveland Clinic group assessed the feasibility and utility of patient-specific physical models corresponding to individual CT scan of patients with liver cirrhosis (Fig. 7.2). They generated multiple cuts of liver physical models corresponding to specific CT cross-sectional slices. They demonstrated that by doing so, identification and spatial relationship of important vascular and biliary structures on imaging studies were made easier (Zein NN, personal communications).

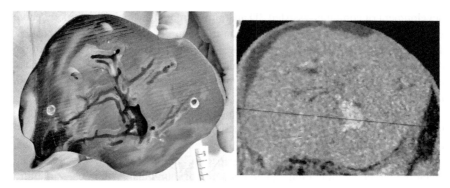

FIGURE 7.2

A cross-sectional cut in a patient-specific 3D printed liver model corresponding to the same slice of CT scan image used as a teaching file for image interpretation.

Liver anatomy and hepatic segments, in particular, represent highly complex anatomical structures with four different types of vascular and biliary conduits that are distributed in an interchanging and staggered manner that commonly thwarts medical students' and young surgeons' efforts to understand surgical anatomy [20,21]. Anatomical corrosion casts have been widely used for such teaching purposes [22–24]. However, the ethical issues associated with their production, the inability of identical reproducibility, the use of original livers in the casting process, and the inability to clearly identify the origin of vessels for each segment by the corrosion method render this technique suboptimal [25]. Although cadaveric models are optimal for training purposes, consistent with our previous discussion, the high costs of preparation in addition to the sociocultural burden make 3D printed organs a very attractive alternative tool to teach gross anatomy. There are now techniques to allow low-cost 3D generated liver models that facilitate medical education, thereby overcoming the shortage of funding that smaller or community institutions may face [26].

A randomized controlled study attempted to assess medical student knowledge acquisition and retention via 3D reconstructed and printed hepatic models [27]. Ninety-two medical students were assigned randomly in each one of the following study arms: (1) traditional anatomic atlas, (2) liver segments without parenchyma, (3) liver segments with transparent parenchyma, and (4) liver ducts with segmental partitions. The study concluded that the 3D printed models improve the teaching effects significantly, while the fourth model seemed to be the most effective one. Another study showed that when 3D printed synthetic models were utilized for simulation in medical education, all of the medical students showed a statistically significant improvement in acquiring and reporting knowledge, as well as their ability to conceptualize critical structures [28].

A cross-sectional study evaluated the use of various 3D printed anatomic models, including one that included a hepatic tumor, in both surgical education and clinical practice [29]. The authors report that 84% of the students and residents believe that such liver cancer models can be particularly important in explaining basic hepatic anatomy, while 90% of the study participants believe that understanding abnormal pathologic anatomy was simplified. Understanding hepatic anatomy in liver tumor models will also facilitate conceptualizing the indications of liver transplantation and liver resection. Additionally, it has been shown that student scores on anatomy tests improved notably after the utilization of 3D printed models [19]. These technological advancements need to be integrated into the medical school curriculum on a much larger and standardized scale.

3D printed models are also useful in patient education (Fig. 7.3). CT- or MRI-derived images are not the easiest or best way to communicate the disease process to patients accurately. 3D printed representations of the patient's liver or other organs can be much more easily understandable for the patient. Patients can easily visualize and understand a malignant entity in their liver through tactile sensation and model manipulation. Additionally, the surgeon can provide a more accurate and detailed explanation about what must be removed by resection or explanted and implanted via transplantation. This becomes a very desirable part of patient and family education as this complex anatomy and surgery becomes much more tangible, touchable, and readily understandable and facilitate the informed consent process. 3D printed organs are especially helpful in the preoperative education of liver donors, who will be able to visualize both the part of their liver that is going to be donated and the remnant tissue. This particular implication is important for expanding the liver graft pool, as more and more people may be eager to donate part of their liver once they obtain a better understanding of the anatomy and operation. It is undebatable that by implementing 3D printing in the everyday clinical practice, the general population will find it easier to entrust their lives in liver transplant surgeons

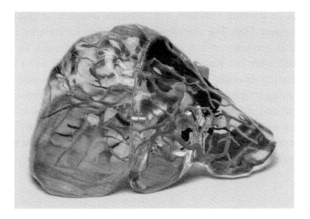

FIGURE 7.3

3D printed liver model of a patient with hepatocellular carcinoma undergoing assessment for surgical resection. The model shows the intended surgical resection line and was used for patient education prior to surgery.

and to gain a better appreciation in the miracle of donating part of their organ. There are data suggesting that via this method, the understanding of hepatic anatomy and physiology increases by 26.4% and 23.6%, respectively, while the understanding of the operation and surgical risks improved by 31.4% and 27.9%, respectively [30]. Last but not least, recent evidence suggests that 1%−2% of Medicare and Medicaid reimbursements may depend on patient satisfaction, which is greatly improved by the increased understanding that 3D printed organs offer [8].

Another aspect of medical teaching is the possibility of training for specific surgical procedures using a patient-specific 3D printed model, especially in complex cases (Fig. 7.3). In this case, physician-in-training can use 3D models for anatomical studies and practice surgical procedures without causing discomfort to an actual patient. 3D simulators could provide a model of the ribs and sternum for proper location of heart sound or placement of ECG leads. Models of the trachea and esophagus could be used in a teaching simulator for the placement of tubes, catheters, or placing a vent. These simulators could be used in the training of nurses and doctors or any other medical-related field. By incorporating 3D technology in training simulators, more accurate representation of the actual procedure task can be obtained. This concept has been tested in a few individual cases including training Urology residents on percutaneous nephrolithotomy [31], a procedure that is associated with significant morbidity during the process to establish access to the renal calyx. In this particular case, a 3D printed training model was created based on CT images of a 65-year-old man presented to the emergency room with renal colic and a 12 mm radio-opaque stone in the lower pole of the left kidney [31]. Investigators used different silicon substances in the process of printing to match the opacity of tissue found in vivo. Trainees involved in this case practiced on the model before performing the actual procedure, which allowed for the anticipation of difficulties inherent to the patient's anatomy [31]. Several additional studies demonstrated the value of physical models in training residents for complex articular fractures [32] and in neurosurgical training [33]. The use of physical models for training in these studies improved surgical proficiency and clinical outcomes, although the models were manufactured and were not based on actual patient anatomy as in the case of 3D printing. 3D printing of more realistic models will likely be associated with an even greater training benefit. Further research is needed in order to assess if the utilization of 3D printed simulation models in education of medical students and surgical residents in transplantation surgery may lead to better quantifiable outcomes and surgical expertise, such as decreased intraoperative complication rates and improved graft survival.

Preoperative surgical planning

There has been an increasing public, governmental, and professional interest in surgical outcomes and means to improve it. A number of studies suggested a relation between the volume of surgeries performed and the rate of complications including mortality, which has been attributed at least in part to the incomplete characterization of anatomical structures in a way to account for individual variations especially in complex surgeries [1,2]. In an effort to optimize outcomes, surgeons used a wide range of preoperative planning techniques in order to improve efficiency, diminish operative time, and ultimately reduce the incidence of surgical complications. Imaging for preoperative planning of high-risk surgical procedures is already widely used, and it provided improved knowledge of anatomical variations [4–6]. Additional approaches beyond standard imaging were more recently introduced to assist in surgical planning and for risk analysis of individual cases, including computer-assisted 3D imaging and the use of surgical models where these techniques provided improved intraoperative orientation. 3D printing has been applied in a limited way as an advanced tool with properties and potential advantages of both 3D imaging and physical surgical models where individual patient's imaging is used to replicate the authentic anatomy of the person to undergo surgery.

Some of earlier use of 3D printing technology in surgical planning happened in the field of Neurosurgery as physicians in these cases encounter some of the most complicated and delicate anatomic structures [34–36]. It is very difficult to fully appreciate complex spinal deformities and obscure structural relationships between cerebral vessels, cranial nerves, and skull base architecture based solely on two-dimensional radiographic images. Any error in navigating this complicated anatomy has potentially devastating consequences. Additionally, the small surgical access field for most neurosurgical surgeries, especially skull base procedures, allows only one surgeon to operate at one time. For these reasons, it would be highly advantageous to create anatomically tailored 3D printed models. These early experiences suggested improved outcome using 3D printed surgical models for preoperative planning in these complex surgeries.

Even though 3D printing technology has many applications and advantages, it cannot be utilized in the emergency setting, at least up to this point in time. The production of a solitary model may take up to 25–40 h, and as such, its use in liver transplantation from donors after cardiac death may exhibit technical issues. On the other hand, in the era of the continually rising need for liver grafts and the tremendous lack of cadaveric livers, living donor liver transplantation (LDLT) constitutes an effective solution to the problem. Western countries are slower to adopt this LDLT in contrast with Asian countries, mostly due to the large supply of deceased donors and the reports of donor morbidity and mortality. These outcomes can, to some degree, be attributed to inadequate preoperative planning regarding the volume of the remnant liver and the anatomical identification of essential structures of the biliary and vascular systems. Therefore, in an attempt to improve donor safety 3D, printed liver models have been evaluated in studies about their application in pre- or even intraoperative planning and simulation.

The first such study was performed at the Cleveland Clinic and validated the use of these models in three liver donors and their three respective recipients (Fig. 7.4) [37]. This was also the first study to assess the accuracy of 3D printed models against the actual human specimens, while the average errors in dimension were less than

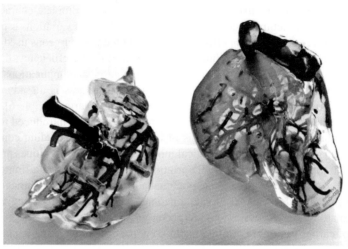

FIGURE 7.4

Patient-specific 3D printed liver model of a healthy liver donor in the setting of a live-donor liver transplant surgery.

1.3 mm for the diameter of vessels and less than 4 mm for the entire graft. The authors highlight the usefulness of this initiative as surgeons appreciated a better understanding of anatomical depth in contrast to the 3D visualization from a 2D screen, while intraoperative navigation was also made possible via real-time manipulation of the models in the operating room (Fig. 7.5). By including data from intraoperative ultrasonography and cholangiography with the use of these models, operative precision may be increased, and operative times may be reduced, hence improving both donor and recipient outcomes [37].

Evidence from another study further solidifies the usefulness of 3D printed hepatic models for preoperative simulation in LDLT [38]. In that case, a 53-year-old man with hepatitis C virus (HCV)-induced cirrhosis, and hepatocellular carcinoma was scheduled to receive his wife's left liver lobe. However, data from 3D images before surgery identified a small-for-size extended left lobe graft, while at the same time, the functional remnant hepatic portion was around one-fifth of her current liver volume. This crested safety concerns. Therefore, a solid 3D printed hepatic model was constructed so that surgeons could improve their spatial perception and decide the appropriate surgical plan. Ultimately, an extended right lobe graft was transplanted from the donor with the hepatic veins being reconstructed ex vivo. Both the donor and the recipient had uncomplicated postoperative courses with decent hepatic function 8 months after transplantation.

Apart from adult patients, LDLT is also a widely accepted therapeutic option for children with end-stage liver disease. Large size is the main issue with LDLT in pediatric patients, especially in small infants as opposed to the concern for small graft size in adults. Hemodynamic imbalance in a large-for-size graft can lead to numerous

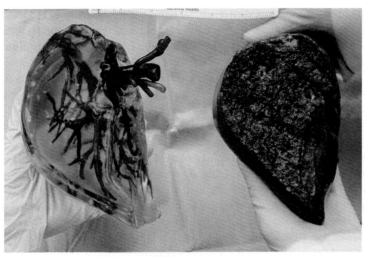

FIGURE 7.5

The use of patient-specific 3D printed liver model for intraoperative navigation in the setting of a live-donor liver transplant surgery.

vessel-related complications, including inadequate perfusion and oxygenation, or even thrombosis of the anastomosed vessels. A large-for-size graft may also be compressed if the abdominal wall is closed in a primary fashion, which is another factor for graft dysfunction. Hence, multiple technical modalities have been utilized from time to time in order to fit part of a large liver into a small abdominal cavity, such as reduced [39], hyperreduced [40], monosegmental [41], and reduced monosegmental liver grafts [42]. The introduction of 3D printing technology can lead to a paradigm shift so that graft size reduction will transition from the subjective "surgeon's experience" into a more objective preplanned method. That way, surgeons will be able to identify vital biliary and vascular structures preoperatively and plan the upcoming procedure with more confidence, fewer complications, and better outcomes. Experience from Japan showed that such a technique was made feasible in an 11-month old female infant, who was about to receive a large-for-size left lateral segment from her father [43]. Graft reduction was performed in situ as planned preoperatively and a 45 g portion was resected, while the remnant portion of the graft was 245 g, and there was no graft- or liver-related complications appreciated in the postoperative course.

Preoperative planning was also made possible via a low-cost, transparent, full-sized 3D printed hepatic model before laparoscopic liver hemihepatectomy for colorectal metastases [44]. The authors of this study report that the overall model costs were less than $150.00, while they used free and open-source software for its fabrication. Therefore, surgeons were able to visualize vascular and biliary structures before taking the patient to the operating room in an inexpensive yet efficient and safe way. Taking into consideration that the era of minimally invasive hepatectomy is here to stay, the donor operation in LDLT is more and more often performed laparoscopically, especially in Asian countries. As a result, fabricating a 3D printed liver model to devise the most appropriate surgical strategy for the laparoscopic graft donation part of LDLT will be of great use and will further improve donor safety and efficiency. Similarly, a group from Poland validated the use of low-cost (100 Euros) 3D printed silicone kidney models for laparoscopic partial nephrectomy simulation and concluded that this method could improve overall surgical outcomes, with a particular decrease in renal ischemia time, while this method can be used in other procedures as well [45].

Multiple studies have evaluated the use of 3D printed hepatic models in the preoperative planning of surgical resection of liver tumors [46,47], including hepatocellular carcinoma [48,49], intrahepatic cholangiocarcinoma [50], hepatoblastoma [51], and liver metastases [52–54]. By involving 3D printed hepatic models in the preoperative strategy of liver surgery, surgeons are able to familiarize and gain experience in performing all types of liver resections, thus improving their technique and skills, and hence achieve lower operative times and lower complication rates. A cross-sectional study showed that 70% and 60% of the surgeons believe that such a model will be useful for both preoperative planning and intraoperative guidance, respectively [29].

A research group from Japan validated the usage of 3D printed organs in surgical navigation and simulation in transplantation surgery. The investigators fabricated two 3D printed kidney and pelvis models from transparent materials based on CT data from patients about to undergo living kidney transplantation [55]. This study showed that surgeons could accurately discuss the operative steps in both the pre- and the intraoperative setting, which facilitates improved understanding of the anatomy and represents a reproducible method of evaluating the surgical operation.

Biliary strictures and cysts form another challenging problem for hepatobiliary surgeons. There is evidence from an Australian group that suggests that 3D printed models of the biliary tree and biliary cysts can be fabricated with high fidelity, while the authors highlight the need for further research in order to decrease the discrepancies between computer-generated images and models [56]. No doubt constructing models for such hepatobiliary pathology will help clarify anatomical associated vascular structures.

3D printing technology can be utilized not only before the liver transplant operation itself but also to deal with its complications, such as portal vein thrombosis. Interventions commonly implemented to resolve this issue include placement of a stent, balloon angioplasty, or surgery as a last resort [57]. A study evaluated the use of 3D printed hollow models of stenosed portal veins to preoperatively simulate endovascular management in a 58-year-old male patient with portal vein stenosis after LDLT [58]. The authors concluded that their model was accurate and precise both in shape and in size, and thus, it should be adopted in clinical practice.

Tissue engineering and bioprinting

The most challenging and potentially complicated use of 3D printing technology today is perhaps in the field of tissue engineering with the intention of regenerating function tissue or ultimately, the fabrication of organs for transplantation. A number of steps to be accomplished and hurdles overcome in order to fabricate a functional 3D tissue resembling human organs including the fact that we are dealing with living cell creating a number of limitations to the use of standard engineering techniques. An integrated system allowing for cell differentiation and for sorting cells based on function locations within a 3D structure is essential. The emergence over the past few years of bioprinters capable of dispensing living cells in a precise position within a 3D structure represents a major advancement in the field although achieving the desired concentration of cells, and a more sustainable growth remain challenges [59]. A wide range of biomaterials (in liquid form or solid-state) has been utilized directly in 3D printers supporting its values in tissue engineering. Another important step to achieve is to be able to create multifunctional scaffolds to meet the structural, mechanical, and nutritional needs of living cells and guide its proliferation and differentiation and adhesion in a way resembling the extracellular matrix seen in native organs [60]. Future advances in fabrication technologies coupled with advances in 3D printing will likely provide the sought after outcome of 3D scaffolds with an internal network of nutrients and materials to satisfy the biological requirement of living cells.

Multiple types of mature differentiated cells have been printed over the past 20 years, while the sources were various organs, including heart, nerves, liver, pancreas, kidney, muscle, bone, or retina. Moreover, the first human amniotic fluid stem cells were 3D printed in 2007 and were subsequently differentiated into functional bone tissue [61]. Many attempts have been made so far to bioprint various types of tissues, including heart valves [62,63], skin [64], cartilage [65], and liver [66]. The Ott laboratory from Massachusetts General Hospital published that decellularized organs, and heart, in particular, can maintain their inherent extracellular matrix and architecture, and function as scaffolds [67]. The subsequent implantation of new myocardial and arterial endothelial cells, while securing the original vascular structures of the organ, led to myocardial contractions and production of heartbeats secondary to cultivation. Optimally, the aim is to fabricate 3D bioprinted tissues and organs from the patient's stem cells, so that they are patient-specific and can be implanted without the need for immunosuppression, thus solving the organ shortage problem. A significant step toward this goal was recently achieved by researchers at Tel Aviv University, who constructed and 3D printed the first human vascularized heart [68].

Bioprinting the liver is an equally challenging process, as its architecture under the microscope is hugely complicated with hepatocytes and the intercalated supporting cells being organized into lobule units in a 3D hexagonal fashion [69]. Bioprinting an artificial liver is difficult, because of the decrease in hepatocyte variability in vitro. When attempting to create a 2D liver model, some of the liver functions cannot be preserved; thus, the 3D printed model is preferred as it can maintain gene expression patterns, metabolic and detoxification functions. Advancements in microtechnology led to a new concept, the "liver-on-a-chip" or "mini-liver," which consists of a microfluidic culture chip embedded with hepatocytes and assists in mimicking the complex in vivo hepatic microenvironment in an in vitro model [70]. The "liver-on-a-chip" model can serve as a tool for drug screening purposes in order to avoid in vivo experiments, which are not optimal for measuring drug-induced hepatotoxicity [71]. Data from a Korean study suggest that human 3D bioprinted liver models in vitro with zonation are even more useful in detecting zonal drug-induced hepatotoxicity by resembling the spatial characteristics of the hexagonal lobular units [72].

The initial step in bioprinting a "mini-liver" was made with the generation of human-induced pluripotent stem cells (hiPSCs) and human embryonic stems cells (hESCs) into alginate hydrogels, which were then differentiated into hepatocyte-like cells (HLCs) with appropriate hepatic morphology and liver marker expression for 21 days [73]. This was followed by the conception of a structure embedded with hepatocytes, human umbilical vein endothelial cells (HUVECs), human lung fibroblasts, and collagen bioink, which could secrete albumin and synthesize urea [74]. The heparin-hydrogel-sandwich method introduced by Foster et al. allowed the in vitro culturing of primary rat hepatocytes, which then had the capability of expressing albumin and cytochrome P450 in high levels for more than 3 weeks [75]. A research team from the University of California, San Diego, produced a 3D bioprinted liver model comprised of hiPSC-derived hepatic progenitor cells (HPCs), human endothelial cells from the umbilical vein, and adipose-derived stem cells organized into the native hexagonal liver lobules [76]. This model showed a betterment in the liver-specific expression of genes, secretion of metabolic products, and induction of cytochrome P450 enzyme system when compared not only to 2D monolayer culture but also the 3D culture of HPCs alone, which can lead to its utilization in early drug screening and disease modeling. The use of alginate [77] or decellularized extracellular matrix [78] as bioinks for the construction of 3D printed HepG2 cell lines highlights that utilizing biocompatible bioinks laden with various cell types in the same culture is of paramount importance due to its ability to increase hepatocyte variability in vitro. Besides, the decellularized hepatic extracellular matrix has been used to re-engineer recellularized hepatic grafts that can mimic in vitro models at a comparable level [79]. Those grafts were able to maintain metabolic enzyme expression, urea synthesis, and albumin secretion at an appropriate level and could be transplanted into rats with insignificant ischemic injury to the hepatocytes. Overall, the generation of biocompatible scaffolds embedded with stem cells seems to be particularly promising and may pave the way for the production of artificial livers that can be transplanted in humans with end-stage liver disease and that will solve the organ shortage issue.

Conclusion

3D printing technology has gained considerable attention over the past years, while more and more research teams worldwide are incorporating it into basic science and clinical research studies. Its implications involve but are not limited to medical and patient education, surgical planning, and bioprinting; the field of hepatobiliary surgery, liver transplantation in general, and LDLT, in particular, is going to be revolutionized by the introduction of 3D printed liver models in everyday clinical practice. The experience we will gain from future studies will lead to a decrease in the cost of these models with their fabrication process being carried out in a timelier manner. Data show that 3D models are becoming more accurate and precise in size and shape and their incorporation in hepatobiliary and transplant surgery will play a vital role in student, resident, and patient education, will improve the outcomes of LDLT, and the upcoming regeneration of whole organs from scaffold laden with stem cells may assist in overcoming the problem of organ shortage. Overall, the constant development in the fabrication of 3D printed models and their incorporation in transplantation will pose a harbinger for the advancement of personalized medicine.

References

[1] Holt PJ, Poloniecki JD, Loftus IM, Michaels JA, Thompson MM. Epidemiological study of the relationship between volume and outcome after abdominal aortic aneurysm surgery in the UK from 2000 to 2005.Epidemiological study of the relationship between volume and outcome after abdominal aortic aneurysm surgery in the UK from 2000 to 2005. Br J Surg 2007;94(4):441–8.

[2] Granger SR, Glasgow RE, Battaglia J, Lee RM, Scaife C, Shrieve DC, et al. Development of a dedicated hepatopancreaticobiliary program in a university hospital system. J Gastrointest Surg 2005;9(7):891–5.

[3] Ellis H. Medicolegal consequences of postoperative intra-abdominal adhesions. J R Soc Med 2001;94(7):331–2.

[4] Royo A, Utrilla C, Carceller F. Surgical management of brainstem-expanding lesions: the role of neuroimaging. Semin Ultrasound CT MR 2013;34(2):153–73. https://doi.org/10.1053/j.sult.2013.01.006.

[5] Sharfuddin A. Imaging evaluation of kidney transplant recipients. Semin Nephrol 2011; 31(3):259–71. https://doi.org/10.1016/j.semnephrol.2011.05.005.

[6] Leipsic J, Yang TH, Min JK. Computed tomographic imaging of transcatheter aortic valve replacement for prediction and prevention of procedural complications. Circ Cardiovasc Imaging 2013;6(4):597–605. https://doi.org/10.1161/circimaging.113.000334.

[7] Mitsouras D, Liacouras P, Imanzadeh A, Giannopoulos AA, Cai T, Kumamaru KK, et al. Medical 3D printing for the radiologist. Radiographics 2015;35(7):1965–88.

[8] Rankin TM, Wormer BA, Miller JD, Giovinco NA, Al Kassis S, Armstrong DG. Image once, print thrice? Three-dimensional printing of replacement parts. Br J Radiol 2018; 91(1083):20170374.

[9] Martelli N, Serrano C, van den Brink H, Pineau J, Prognon P, Borget I, et al. Advantages and disadvantages of 3-dimensional printing in surgery: a systematic review. Surgery 2016;159(6):1485–500.

[10] Randazzo M, Pisapia JM, Singh N, Thawani JP. 3D printing in neurosurgery: a systematic review. Surg Neurol Int 2016;7(Suppl. 33):S801–9.

[11] Bartel T, Rivard A, Jimenez A, Mestres CA, Muller S. Medical three-dimensional printing opens up new opportunities in cardiology and cardiac surgery. Eur Heart J 2018; 39(15):1246–54.

[12] Aziz MA, McKenzie JC, Wilson JS, Cowie RJ, Ayeni SA, Dunn BK. The human cadaver in the age of biomedical informatics. Anat Rec 2002;269(1):20—32.

[13] Jones DG, Whitaker MI. Anatomy's use of unclaimed bodies: reasons against continued dependence on an ethically dubious practice. Clin Anat 2012;25(2):246—54. https://doi.org/10.1002/ca.21223. Epub 2011 Jul 28.

[14] Khalil MK, Paas F, Johnson TE, Payer AF. Interactive and dynamic visualizations in teaching and learning of anatomy: a cognitive load perspective. Anat Rec B New Anat 2005;286(1):8—14.

[15] Nguyen N, Wilson TD. A head in virtual reality: development of a dynamic head and neck model. Anat Sci Educ 2009;2(6):294—301. https://doi.org/10.1002/ase.115.

[16] Levinson AJ, Weaver B, Garside S, McGinn H, Norman GR. Virtual reality and brain anatomy: a randomised trial of e-learning instructional designs. Med Educ 2007;41(5):495—501.

[17] Khalil MK, Mansour MM, Wilhite DR. Evaluation of cognitive loads imposed by traditional paper-based and innovative computer-based instructional strategies. J Vet Med Educ 2010;37(4):353—7. https://doi.org/10.3138/jvme.37.4.353.

[18] Rengier F, Häfner MF, Unterhinninghofen R, Nawrotzki R, Kirsch J, Kauczor HU, et al. Integration of interactive three-dimensional image post-processing software into undergraduate radiology education effectively improves diagnostic skills and visual-spatial ability. Eur J Radiol 2013;82(8):1366—71. https://doi.org/10.1016/j.ejrad.2013.01.010.

[19] Preece D, Williams SB, Lam R, Weller R. "Let's get physical": advantages of a physical model over 3D computer models and textbooks in learning imaging anatomy. Anat Sci Educ 2013;6(4):216—24. https://doi.org/10.1002/ase.1345.

[20] Farid SG, Prasad KR, Morris-Stiff G. Operative terminology and post-operative management approaches applied to hepatic surgery: trainee perspectives. World J Gastrointest Surg 2013;5(5):146—55.

[21] Oliveira DA, Feitosa RQ, Correia MM. Segmentation of liver, its vessels and lesions from CT images for surgical planning. Biomed Eng Online 2011;10:30.

[22] Ursic M, Ravnik D, Hribernik M, Pecar J, Butinar J, Fazarinc G. Gross anatomy of the portal vein and hepatic artery ramifications in dogs: corrosion cast study. Anat Histol Embryol 2007;36(2):83—7.

[23] Ursic M, Vrecl M, Fazarinc G. Corrosion cast study of the canine hepatic veins. Folia Morphol 2014;73(4):475—81.

[24] Nemeth K, Deshpande R, Mathe Z, Szuak A, Kiss M, Korom C, et al. Extrahepatic arteries of the human liver - anatomical variants and surgical relevancies. Transpl Int 2015;28(10):1216—26.

[25] Li J, Nie L, Li Z, Lin L, Tang L, Ouyang J. Maximizing modern distribution of complex anatomical spatial information: 3D reconstruction and rapid prototype production of anatomical corrosion casts of human specimens. Anat Sci Educ 2012;5(6):330—9.

[26] Javan R, Herrin D, Tangestanipoor A. Understanding spatially complex segmental and branch anatomy using 3D printing: liver, lung, prostate, coronary arteries, and circle of Willis. Acad Radiol 2016;23(9):1183—9.

[27] Kong X, Nie L, Zhang H, Wang Z, Ye Q, Tang L, et al. Do 3D printing models improve anatomical teaching about hepatic segments to medical students? A randomized controlled study. World J Surg 2016;40(8):1969—76.

[28] Costello JP, Olivieri LJ, Krieger A, Thabit O, Marshall MB, Yoo S-J, et al. Utilizing three-dimensional printing technology to assess the feasibility of high-fidelity synthetic

ventricular septal defect models for simulation in medical education. World J Pediatr Congenit Heart Surg 2014;5(3):421−6.

[29] Jones DB, Sung R, Weinberg C, Korelitz T, Andrews R. Three-dimensional modeling may improve surgical education and clinical practice. Surg Innov 2016;23(2):189−95.

[30] Yang T, Tan T, Yang J, Pan J, Hu C, Li J, et al. The impact of using three-dimensional printed liver models for patient education. J Int Med Res 2018;46(4):1570−8.

[31] Bruyère F, Leroux C, Brunereau L, Lermusiaux P. Rapid prototyping model for percu-taneous nephrolithotomy training. J Endourol 2008;22(1):91−6. https://doi.org/10.1089/end.2007.0025.

[32] Yehyawi TM, Thomas TP, Ohrt GT, Marsh JL, Karam MD, Brown TD, et al. A simulation trainer for complex articular fracture surgery. J Bone Joint Surg Am 2013;95(13):e92. https://doi.org/10.2106/JBJS.L.00554.

[33] Jabbour P, Chalouhi N. Simulation-based neurosurgical training for the presigmoid approach with a physical model. Neurosurgery 2013;73(Suppl. 1):81−4. https://doi.org/10.1227/NEU.0000000000000090.

[34] Spottiswoode BS, van den Heever DJ, Chang Y, Engelhardt S, Du Plessis S, Nicolls F, et al. Preoperative three-dimensional model creation of magnetic resonance brain im-ages as a tool to assist neurosurgical planning. Stereotact Funct Neurosurg 2013;91(3):162−9. https://doi.org/10.1159/000345264.

[35] Waran V, Pancharatnam D, Thambinayagam HC, Raman R, Rathinam AK, Balakrishnan YK, et al. The utilization of cranial models created using rapid prototyp-ing techniques in the development of models for navigation training. J Neurol Surg A Cent Eur Neurosurg 2014;75(1):12−5. https://doi.org/10.1055/s-0032-1330960.

[36] Aydin HE, Kaya I, Aydin N, Kizmazoglu C, Karakoc F, Yurt H, Hüsemoglu RB. Impor-tance of three-dimensional modeling in cranioplasty. J Craniofac Surg 2019;30:713−5.

[37] Zein NN, Hanouneh IA, Bishop PD, Samaan M, Eghtesad B, Quintini C, et al. Three-dimensional print of a liver for preoperative planning in living donor liver transplantation. Liver Transplant Off Publ Am Assoc Study Liver Dis Int Liver Trans-plant Soc 2013;19(12):1304−10.

[38] Baimakhanov Z, Soyama A, Takatsuki M, Hidaka M, Hirayama T, Kinoshita A, et al. Pre-operative simulation with a 3-dimensional printed solid model for one-step reconstruction of multiple hepatic veins during living donor liver transplantation. In: Liver transplanta-tion , vol. 21. United States: official publication of the American Association for the Study of Liver Diseases and the International Liver Transplantation Society; 2015. p. 266−8.

[39] Broelsch CE, Emond JC, Thistlethwaite JR, Whitington PF, Zucker AR, Baker AL, et al. Liver transplantation, including the concept of reduced-size liver transplants in children. Ann Surg 1988;208(4):410−20.

[40] Thomas N, Thomas G, Verran D, Stormon M, O'Loughlin E, Shun A. Liver transplan-tation in children with hyper-reduced grafts - a single-center experience. Pediatr Trans-plant 2010;14(3):426−30.

[41] Kasahara M, Uryuhara K, Kaihara S, Kozaki K, Fujimoto Y, Ogura Y, et al. Monoseg-mental living donor liver transplantation. Transplant Proc 2003;35(4):1425−6.

[42] Ogawa K, Kasahara M, Sakamoto S, Ito T, Taira K, Oike F, et al. Living donor liver transplantation with reduced monosegments for neonates and small infants. Transplan-tation 2007;83(10):1337−40.

[43] Soejima Y, Taguchi T, Sugimoto M, Hayashida M, Yoshizumi T, Ikegami T, et al. Three-dimensional printing and biotexture modeling for preoperative simulation in living donor liver transplantation for small infants. Liver transplantation , vol. 22. United

States: official publication of the American Association for the Study of Liver Diseases and the International Liver Transplantation Society; 2016. p. 1610–4.

[44] Witowski JS, Pedziwiatr M, Major P, Budzynski A. Cost-effective, personalized, 3D-printed liver model for preoperative planning before laparoscopic liver hemihepatectomy for colorectal cancer metastases. Int J Comput Assist Radiol Surg 2017;12(12): 2047–54.

[45] Golab A, Smektala T, Kaczmarek K, Stamirowski R, Hrab M, Slojewski M. Laparoscopic partial nephrectomy supported by training involving personalized silicone replica poured in three-dimensional printed casting mold. J Laparoendosc Adv Surg Tech 2017;27(4):420–2.

[46] Madurska MJ, Poyade M, Eason D, Rea P, Watson AJM. Development of a patient-specific 3d-printed liver model for preoperative planning. Surg Innov 2017;24(2): 145–50.

[47] Oshiro Y, Mitani J, Okada T, Ohkohchi N. A novel three-dimensional print of liver vessels and tumors in hepatectomy. Surg Today [Internet] 2017;47(4):521–4. Available from: https://doi.org/10.1007/s00595-016-1383-8.

[48] Xiang N, Fang C, Fan Y, Yang J, Zeng N, Liu J, et al. Application of liver three-dimensional printing in hepatectomy for complex massive hepatocarcinoma with rare variations of portal vein: preliminary experience. Int J Clin Exp Med 2015;8(10): 18873–8.

[49] Perica E, Sun Z. Patient-specific three-dimensional printing for pre-surgical planning in hepatocellular carcinoma treatment. Quant Imaging Med Surg 2017;7(6):668–77.

[50] Takagi K, Nanashima A, Abo T, Arai J, Matsuo N, Fukuda T, et al. Three-dimensional printing model of liver for operative simulation in perihilar cholangiocarcinoma. Hepato-Gastroenterology 2014;61(136):2315–6.

[51] Souzaki R, Kinoshita Y, Ieiri S, Hayashida M, Koga Y, Shirabe K, et al. Three-dimensional liver model based on preoperative CT images as a tool to assist in surgical planning for hepatoblastoma in a child. Pediatr Surg Int [Internet] 2015;31(6):593–6. Available from: https://doi.org/10.1007/s00383-015-3709-9.

[52] Igami T, Nakamura Y, Hirose T, Ebata T, Yokoyama Y, Sugawara G, et al. Application of a three-dimensional print of a liver in hepatectomy for small tumors invisible by intraoperative ultrasonography: preliminary experience. World J Surg [Internet] 2014; 38(12):3163–6. Available from: https://doi.org/10.1007/s00268-014-2740-7.

[53] Leng S, Chen B, Vrieze T, Kuhlmann J, Yu L, Alexander A, et al. Construction of realistic phantoms from patient images and a commercial three-dimensional printer. J Med Imaging (Bellingham, Wash) 2016;3(3):33501.

[54] Choi YR, Kim JH, Park SJ, Hur BY, Han JK. Therapeutic response assessment using 3D ultrasound for hepatic metastasis from colorectal cancer: application of a personalized, 3D-printed tumor model using CT images. PLoS One 2017;12(8):e0182596.

[55] Kusaka M, Sugimoto M, Fukami N, Sasaki H, Takenaka M, Anraku T, et al. Initial experience with a tailor-made simulation and navigation program using a 3-D printer model of kidney transplantation surgery. Transplant Proc 2015;47(3):596–9.

[56] Allan A, Kealley C, Squelch A, Wong YH, Yeong CH, Sun Z. Patient-specific 3D printed model of biliary ducts with congenital cyst. Quant Imaging Med Surg 2019; 9(1):86–93.

[57] Tirumani SH, Shanbhogue AKP, Vikram R, Prasad SR, Menias CO. Imaging of the porta hepatis: spectrum of disease. Radiographics 2014;34(1):73–92.

[58] Takao H, Amemiya S, Shibata E, Ohtomo K. Three-dimensional printing of hollow portal vein stenosis models: a feasibility study. In: Journal of vascular and interventional radiology, vol. 27. United States: JVIR; 2016. p. 1755—8.

[59] Mironov V, Kasyanov V, Markwald RR. Organ printing: from bioprinter to organ biofabrication line. Curr Opin Biotechnol 2011;22(5):667—73. https://doi.org/10.1016/j.copbio.2011.02.006.

[60] Lee M, Wu BM. In computer-aided tissue engineering. In: Methods in molecular biology by michael A.K. Liebschner. Springer Science and Business Media; 2012.

[61] De Coppi P, Bartsch GJ, Siddiqui MM, Xu T, Santos CC, Perin L, et al. Isolation of amniotic stem cell lines with potential for therapy. Nat Biotechnol 2007;25(1):100—6.

[62] Duan B, Hockaday LA, Kang KH, Butcher JT. 3D bioprinting of heterogeneous aortic valve conduits with alginate/gelatin hydrogels. J Biomed Mater Res A 2013;101(5):1255—64.

[63] Duan B, Kapetanovic E, Hockaday LA, Butcher JT. Three-dimensional printed trileaflet valve conduits using biological hydrogels and human valve interstitial cells. Acta Biomater 2014;10(5):1836—46.

[64] Nahmias Y, Arneja A, Tower TT, Renn MJ, Odde DJ. Cell patterning on biological gels via cell spraying through a mask. Tissue Eng 2005;11(5—6):701—8.

[65] Chen H, Wu D, Yang H, Guo K. Clinical use of 3D printing guide plate in posterior lumbar pedicle screw fixation. Med Sci Monit 2015;21:3948—54.

[66] Wang X, Yu X, Yan Y, Zhang R. Liver tissue responses to gelatin and gelatin/chitosan gels. J Biomed Mater Res A 2008;87(1):62—8.

[67] Ott HC, Matthiesen TS, Goh S-K, Black LD, Kren SM, Netoff TI, et al. Perfusion-decellularized matrix: using nature's platform to engineer a bioartificial heart. Nat Med 2008;14(2):213—21.

[68] Noor N, Shapira A, Edri R, Gal I, Wertheim L, Dvir T. 3D printing of personalized thick and perfusable cardiac patches and hearts. Adv Sci [Internet] 2019. 1900344. Available from: https://onlinelibrary.wiley.com/doi/abs/10.1002/advs.201900344.

[69] Alkhouri N, Zein NN. Three-dimensional printing and pediatric liver disease. Curr Opin Pediatr 2016;28(5):626—30.

[70] Yoon No D, Lee K-H, Lee J, Lee S-H. 3D liver models on a microplatform: well-defined culture, engineering of liver tissue and liver-on-a-chip. Lab Chip 2015;15(19):3822—37.

[71] Griffith LG, Swartz MA. Capturing complex 3D tissue physiology in vitro. Nat Rev Mol Cell Biol 2006;7(3):211—24.

[72] Ahn J, Ahn J-H, Yoon S, Nam YS, Son M-Y, Oh J-H. Human three-dimensional in vitro model of hepatic zonation to predict zonal hepatotoxicity. J Biol Eng 2019;13:22.

[73] Faulkner-Jones A, Fyfe C, Cornelissen D-J, Gardner J, King J, Courtney A, et al. Bioprinting of human pluripotent stem cells and their directed differentiation into hepatocyte-like cells for the generation of mini-livers in 3D. Biofabrication 2015;7(4):44102.

[74] Lee JW, Choi Y-J, Yong W-J, Pati F, Shim J-H, Kang KS, et al. Development of a 3D cell printed construct considering angiogenesis for liver tissue engineering. Biofabrication 2016;8(1):15007.

[75] Foster E, You J, Siltanen C, Patel D, Haque A, Anderson L, et al. Heparin hydrogel sandwich cultures of primary hepatocytes. Eur Polym J [Internet] 2015;72:726—35. Available from: http://www.sciencedirect.com/science/article/pii/S0014305714004741.

[76] Ma X, Qu X, Zhu W, Li Y-S, Yuan S, Zhang H, et al. Deterministically patterned bio-mimetic human iPSC-derived hepatic model via rapid 3D bioprinting. Proc Natl Acad Sci U S A 2016;113(8):2206−11.

[77] Jeon H, Kang K, Park SA, Kim WD, Paik SS, Lee S-H, et al. Generation of multilayered 3D structures of HepG2 cells using a bio-printing technique. Gut Liver 2017;11(1): 121−8.

[78] Lee H, Han W, Kim H, Ha D-H, Jang J, Kim BS, et al. Development of liver decellularized extracellular matrix bioink for three-dimensional cell printing-based liver tissue engineering. Biomacromolecules 2017;18(4):1229−37.

[79] Uygun BE, Soto-Gutierrez A, Yagi H, Izamis M-L, Guzzardi MA, Shulman C, et al. Organ reengineering through development of a transplantable recellularized liver graft using decellularized liver matrix. Nat Med 2010;16(7):814−20.

3D printing in cardiac surgery

Kyriakos Anastasiadis, MD, PhD, FETCS, FCCP,
Georgios I. Tagarakis, MD, PhD, FETCS
Department of Cardiothoracic Surgery, Aristotle University of Thessaloniki, AHEPA University
Hospital, Thessaloniki, Greece

The technology of three-dimensional printing was invented in 1983 by Chuck Hull, an American physicist and engineer [1,2]. He was the first to conceive the idea that the induction of light over multiple thin plastic layers positioned over each other would be able to lead to the construction of three-dimensional objects. Hull came up with the idea while working with ultraviolet light to harden tabletop coatings. In his original concept, a computer-guided beam of ultraviolet light is directed over liquid photopolymer transforming it into plastic. The idea is not just restricted to liquids but can be applied to all substances that have the capacity to alter their condition or become solidified. His invention is usually described by the terms 3D printing, stereolithography, or additive manufacturing. In a few words, 3D printing is a new technology aimed at transforming digital images to physical objects. In 1986, Hull founded in California the enterprise 3D Systems, which has since then become the pioneer for the developments in 3D printing worldwide.

As far as the procedure of 3D printing is concerned, this includes various stages [3]. At first, a computer model design for the specific production is created, based on the application of specialized software. Afterward, the 3D printer is loaded with the production material. This is usually plastic, but can include a variety of other materials, such as metal, glass, sand, clay, and biomaterials. Finally, the process of ejection takes place, ending to the extraction of the requested product from the printer. Quite often, some extra final steps of processing are necessary in order to freeze the produced object and clean it as well as detach it from the printer or from supporting structures.

The 3D printers can vary substantially in size and shape depending on their application. Generally, the progress in related technology constantly produces faster, cheaper, and more sizable models. Lately, stereolithography which is a laser-based 3D printing technology that uses UV-sensitive liquid resins is one of the most widely used rapid prototyping technologies. The current application of 3D printing technology in science and human activity encompasses various fields: aerospace engineering, mechanical engineering, cosmetology, medicine, dentistry, etc. The main advantage of this form of production is the ability to construct objects based on individualized needs, at low cost and beyond the standard industrialized

3D Printing: Applications in Medicine and Surgery. https://doi.org/10.1016/B978-0-323-66164-5.00008-8

lines of production. Since this technique opens the possibility of manufacturing highly specialized products to a broad spectrum of customers, it is already considered as a revolution in science and technology as well as in industry and commerce.

Cardiac surgery
Evolution of cardiac surgery

Cardiac Surgery is the medical discipline dealing with the surgical treatment of congenital and acquired diseases of the heart and great vessels. Among the most common procedures within the specialty are coronary artery bypass grafting; aortic, mitral, and tricuspid valve surgery (replacement and repair); and surgery on the thoracic aorta as well as various procedures for heart anomalies. Furthermore, the full spectrum of the specialty comprises minimally invasive, endoscopic, endovascular, and robotic procedures.

Francisco Romero [4], a Catalonian physician, became the first heart surgeon when he performed an open pericardiostomy to treat a pericardial effusion in 1801. He presented his work at the Society of the School of Medicine in Paris in 1815, but the procedure was considered too aggressive and his work was silenced for many years. Almost a 100 years later, in 1896, Ludwig Rehn [5], a German surgeon, repaired a stab wound to the heart by direct suture, thus starting the era of heart surgery. The first half cycle was the period of closed heart surgery when mainly congenital diseases of the heart were treated surgically. It was John Gibbon in 1953 [6], an American heart surgeon, who managed to perform the first successful open heart operation with the use of a heart-lung machine. Introduction and wide use of this machine, called thereafter extracorporeal circulation, enabled cardiac surgery to expand its potential into the heart (open heart surgery) and hence deal thoroughly with the congenital as well as all acquired heart diseases, i.e., coronary artery disease, valve diseases, transplantation, aortic surgery, etc. Thus, cardiac surgery became a routine surgery. Nowadays, it is estimated that over 1 million heart operations are performed worldwide annually. This number clearly shows both the progress of the specialty, as well as its impact on the current health status of the general population internationally.

There are not many specialties so tightly linked to technology as cardiac surgery. The extracorporeal circulation machine, one of the highest technologies used, substitutes the pumping action of the heart and the respiratory function of the lungs during the surgical procedure. Hi-tech monitoring devices are employed in order to control perfusion intraoperatively. Furthermore, high-resolution cardiac computed tomography and cardiac magnetic resonance are often used for the preoperative planning of cardiac procedures. Pacemakers, prosthetic valves, mechanical assist devices, and artificial hearts are all products of advanced technology related to heart surgery. This reality, along with the fact that the cardiovascular system has a lot of variations, comprises the rationale for the necessity of preoperative study of three-dimensional models and subsequent design of the surgical procedure in such a wide range pathology. Thus, cardiac surgery represents one of the fields where 3D printing is expected to contribute to the progress of the specialty.

Applications of 3D printing in cardiac surgery
Teaching aid
A primary application of 3D printing is to produce models for anatomic teaching or demonstration [1,7]. Thus, similarly to the plastic heart models familiar to most health care professionals, a 3D-printed model can rapidly convey a complex anatomic arrangement, but has the added value of also depicting patient-specific anatomic pathology. Such models can be instructional for the teaching of medical professionals about normal and abnormal structural relationships and can also be used to explain to the public or the patients the anatomy and physiology of cardiovascular disorders. Patient-specific models of congenital heart are used for training of younger physicians and nurses. Examples include instructional models depicting congenital heart defects, valve stenosis, and catheter-based valve implantation or repair procedures. Increasingly, these 3D models can be constructed with particular colors, variable material hardness, and even layered texturing, if needed, to depict sophisticated or unusual cardiovascular pathology.

Procedure planning
Complex procedures related to congenital heart defects, or to the reconstruction of valves or the aorta, require meticulous preoperative study and planning [8]. Patient-specific 3D printing models created based on the information provided by computed tomography or magnetic resonance imaging can be an invaluable tool in the hands of the heart surgical team planning their corrective intervention of the congenital or acquired cardiovascular anomalies. As a consequence, the procedure may be much easier understood, discussed, thoroughly studied, and finally accurately planned on a three-dimensional model closely resembling the anatomical conditions of the affected area. The possible therapeutic alternatives and the outcome of the proposed corrections can also be visualized and reproduced based on a 3D model.

It seems that the reconstruction of a patient's coronary anatomy through 3D printing is another field of application of this new technology. In a recent publication, Javan et al. [9] demonstrated that a variety of 3D print models were ideal for coronary visualization. The coronary artery tree can be depicted in detail by gated CT methods, so that all stenotic or occlusive areas can be clearly visualized, aiding to the better planning of the procedure. If the coronary tree is 3D printed based on the diastolic phase, useful information about the epicardial coronary perfusion can be gained. In addition, such models can provide a reference standard for testing of novel diagnostic measurements (e.g., CT-derived fractional flow reserve, FFR) against a controlled in vitro forward flow gold standard. Kolli et al. [10] published a related article presenting their experience on the 3D modeling of coronary arteries with stenotic lesions ranging from 30% to 70%. The stenotic lesions were correlated with absolute decreases in FFR ranging from 0.03 to 0.2, respectively. Their work demonstrates how 3D printing can provide useful information in the study of coronary flow in a quantitative as well as systematic manner.

Maragiannis et al. [11,12] reported their work on 3D-based models created to study the characteristics of patients suffering from severe aortic valve stenosis. They demonstrated that 3D-printed models can replicate both the anatomic and functional properties of severe degenerative aortic valve stenosis. These full-scale models of specific patient anatomy and valve function can be created by combining the technologies of high spatial resolution ECG-gated CT, computer-aided design software, and fused dual-material 3D printing. The development of patient-specific models that accurately replicate both anatomic and functional characteristics may have multiple near-future applications. Recently, Ong et al. [13] presented a case report of a disease with a very complex anatomy comprising a right-sided aortic arch, a Kommerell's diverticulum and an aberrant left subclavian artery. This patient, with an otherwise difficult to interpret intraoperatively anatomic pathology, underwent successful surgical repair with the aid of a printed patient-specific 3D model before surgery, which served as a surgical guide to select the size of graft and to decide on the section to resect; hence, 3D printing can reduce operative time and enhance the optimum result of the correction. Scanlan et al. [14] presented their work on pediatric valve models created based on 3D printing technology: leaflets of a pediatric mitral valve, a tricuspid valve in a hypoplastic left heart syndrome, and complete atrioventricular canal valve were segmented from ultrasound images; a custom software was developed to automatically generate molds for each valve based on the segmentation; these molds were 3D printed and used to make silicone valve models, which were designed with cylindrical rims of different sizes surrounding the leaflets, to show the outline of the valve and add rigidity. Pediatric cardiac surgeons practiced suturing on the models and evaluated them for use as surgical planning and training tools. As a result, five out of six surgeons reported that the valve models would be very useful as planning or training tools for cardiac surgery. In this first iteration of valve models, leaflets were felt to be unrealistically thick or stiff compared to real patient leaflets. A thin tube rim was preferred for valve flexibility. The investigators concluded that further improvements should be made based on the surgeons' feedback. With this perfect example, it is obviously highlighted that due to the difficulty in fully understanding the complex, three-dimensional anatomy of the congenital heart disorders, pediatric cardiac surgery is one of the main fields where stereolithography has already and is expected to obtain even more applications.

Sodian et al. [15,16] published their work on stereolithographic creation of 3D models of patients referred for redo operation of aortic valve replacement due to severe valve stenosis with coronary artery bypass grafting in their past medical history. With the produced models, both the coronary anatomy as well as the structure of adhesive precardiac tissues could be depicted in detail. The models were sterilized and brought into the operating theater where they proved to be of great assistance for the surgeons during the procedure, helping them to avoid the injury of the native heart structures, as well as the patent bypass grafts. In another application of stereolithography, the authors used 3D-replicas in an HIV positive patient who had been operated for a type A dissection, and who had an aortic arch pseudoaneurysm with a slit-shaped entrance hole located anteriorly to the implanted supra-aortic vessels. Computed tomography data were obtained and a lifelike replica of the complex pathology of the aorta using a rapid prototyping machine was fabricated. After careful examination of the model, a custom-made occluder device for interventional closure of the leakage was constructed. Al Jabbari et al. [17] reported their experience with stereolithography to create models depicting the anatomy of patients suffering from complex cardiac tumors, with detailed reconstruction of the main tumor characteristics: size, location, and extension. This information also proved to be very helpful in the preoperative planning of the surgical procedures.

Device innovation and testing

Applications of 3D printing technology in the field of device innovation and testing are already in clinical practice. Such an example is the case of transcatheter mitral valve replacement devices. The development of these devices has been slower and more challenging than the development of other similar technologies, like Mitral-Clip or transaortic valve replacement technologies [18−20]. Although highly specialized software programs like 3Dimensio offer important data in regard to the anatomical properties of the diseased region, a 3D-based physical model may additively offer further useful information. Thus, it may show the impact of the application of the device on the diseased mitral valve area as well as the impact of the diseased area, especially in cases of highly calcified lesions to the device itself. Related models have already been created aiming at the testing and improvement of novel devices.

Production of implantable devices, conduits, and prosthesis

Initially, the variety of products resulting from the procedure of 3D printing was really limited, deriving mostly from rigid raw materials. Meanwhile, the development of technology has created a wider margin of materials favorable for 3D-use, some of them cheap and more flexible [21,22]. In order to simulate the properties of myocardial or vascular tissue, further advances have to be made, in such a way that the production of anatomical heart or vascular parts could be implantable. However, based on the aforementioned continuous improvement of materials and technology progress, favorable results are expected soon.

Conclusions

The complexity of anatomic disorders in heart surgery, as well as the dynamic pathophysiology related to them, poses many problems in understanding, planning, and performing surgical procedures. In addition, many devices applied in heart surgery, and especially in hybrid or endovascular procedures, need to be individually prepared for the patient. Such issues may be facilitated by 3D printing. This chapter presents contemporary advancements in bioengineering, along these lines, that are already applied in heart surgery. Improvements on the field and the related technology will further lower the cost and increase the efficiency of the production. In any case, 3D printing is undoubtedly one of the most promising fields in modern technology, while cardiac surgery is expected to benefit a lot from this progress.

References

[1] Farooqi KM, Sengupta PP. Echocardiography and three-dimensional printing: sound ideas to touch a heart. J Am Soc Echocardiogr 2015;28:398−403.

[2] U.S. Patent 4,575,330. Apparatus for production of three-dimensional objects by stereolithography.

[3] Vukicevic M, Mosadegh B, Min JK, Little S3. Cardiac 3D printing and its future directions. JACC Cardiovasc Imag 2017;10:171−84.

[4] Aris A. Francisco Romero, the first heart surgeon. Ann Thorac Surg 1997;64:870−1.

[5] Werner OJ, Sohns C, Popov AF, Haskamp J, Schmitto JD. Ludwig Rehn (1849-1930): the German surgeon who performed the worldwide first successful cardiac operation. J Med Biogr 2012;20:32−4.

[6] Castillo JG, Silvay G, John H, Gibbon Jr., and the 60th anniversary of the first successful heart-lung machine. J Cardiothorac Vasc Anesth 2013;27:203−7.

[7] Kiraly L, Tofeig M, Jha NK, Talo H. Three-dimensional printed prototypes refine the anatomy of post-modified Norwood-1 complex aortic arch obstruction and allow pre-surgical simulation of the repair. Interact Cardiovasc Thorac Surg 2016;22:238−40.

[8] Vukicevic M, Maragiannis D, Jackson M, Little SH. Functional evaluation of a patient-specific 3D printed model of aortic regurgitation (abstr) circulation. F. 2015. p. 132.

[9] Javan R, Herrin D, Tangestanipoor A. Understanding spatially complex segmental and branch anatomy using 3D printing: liver, lung, prostate, coronary arteries, and Circle of Willis. Acad Radiol 2016;23:1183−9.

[10] Kolli KK, Min JK, Ha S, Soohoo H, Xiong G. Effect of varying hemodynamic and vascular conditions on fractional flow reserve: an in vitro study. J Am Heart Assoc 2016;5(7):e003634.

[11] Maragiannis D, Jackson MS, Igo SR, Chang SM, Zoghbi WA, Little SH. Functional 3D printed patient-specific modeling of severe aortic stenosis. J Am Coll Cardiol 2014;64: 1066−8.

[12] Maragiannis D, Jackson MS, Igo SR, et al. Replicating patient-specific severe aortic valve stenosis with functional 3D modeling. Circ Cardiovasc Imag 2015;8:e003626.

[13] Ong SC, Narutoshi H. The use of 3D printing in cardiac surgery. J Thorac Dis 2017;9: 2301−2.

[14] Scanlan AB, Nguyen AV, Ilina A, et al. Comparison of 3D echocardiogram-derived 3D printed valve models to molded models for simulated repair of pediatric atrioventricular valves. Pediatr Cardiol 2018;39:538−47.

[15] Sodian R, Schmauss D, Markert M, et al. Three-dimensional printing creates models for surgical planning of aortic valve replacement after previous coronary bypass grafting. Ann Thorac Surg 2008;85:2105−8.

[16] Sodian R, Schmauss D, Schmitz C, et al. 3-dimensional printing of models to create custom-made devices for coil embolization of an anastomotic leak after aortic arch replacement. Ann Thorac Surg 2009;88:974−8.

[17] Al Jabbari O, Abu Saleh WK, Patel AP, Igo SR, Reardon MJ. Use of three-dimensional models to assist in the resection of malignant cardiac tumors. J Card Surg 2016;31: 581−3.

[18] Vukicevic M, Puperi DS, Jane Grande-Allen K, Little SH. 3D printed modeling of the mitral valve for catheter-based structural interventions. Ann Biomed Eng 2016;44: 3432.

[19] Kheradvar A, Groves EM, Simmons CA, et al. Emerging trends in heart valve engineering: Part III. Novel technologies for mitral valve repair and replacement. Ann Biomed Eng 2015;43:858−70.

[20] Blanke P, Naoum C, Webb J, et al. Multimodality imaging in the context of transcatheter mitral valve replacement: establishing consensus among modalities and disciplines. JACC Cardiovasc Imag 2015;8:1191−208.

[21] Yang DH, Kang JW, Kim N, Song JK, Lee JW, Lim TH. Myocardial 3-dimensional printing for septal myectomy guidance in a patient with obstructive hypertrophic cardiomyopathy. Circulation 2015;132:300−1.

[22] Wang K, Zhao Y, Chang Y, et al. Controlling the mechanical behavior of dual-material 3D printed meta-materials for patient-specific tissue-mimicking phantoms. Mater Des 2016;90:704−12.

3D printing in vascular surgery

Georgios Koufopoulos, MD[1]**, Konstantinos Skarentzos, MS**[1]**,
Efstratios Georgakarakos, MD, MSc, PhD**[2]

[1]*Medical School, Democritus University of Thrace, Alexandroupolis, Greece;* [2]*Assistant Professor
of Vascular Surgery, Department of Vascular Surgery, Medical School, University Hospital of
Alexandroupolis, Democritus University of Thrace, Alexandroupolis, Greece*

3D printing for preoperative planning

3D printing has a major role in preoperative assessment and simulation of surgical and endovascular procedures. 3D models are constructed to aid clinical doctors and scientists understand the anatomy and disorders of the thoracic and abdominal aorta [1–6].

Ho et al. indicated that vessel diameters acquired from pre-3D printing computed tomography (CT) images and images obtained from model's CT scan presented only minor differences within 1 mm error, ensuring the highest anatomical accuracy of the rapid prototype [7]. Furthermore, the 3D printed models used in the preoperative planning over the last 5 years have decreased the procedural time and complication rates with regard to surgical management of abdominal aortic aneurysms (AAA) and aortic dissections. The use of 3D printing has been also described in preoperative planning of portosystemic shunt closure devices [8].

3D printing has been used for preoperational planning of endovascular treatment for various aortic stenosis pathologies, such as hypoplasia [9], aortic valve stenosis [10,11], pulmonary valve stenosis [12], and internal carotid artery stenosis [13], but also for portal vein stenosis [14]. Aortic dissection has been shown to be an aortic pathology that 3D printed models could enable direct visualization and assessment of anatomical features, regarding the size and shape of true and false lumens, something which should lead in the best clinical decision making and medical treatment [7]. Notably, the greatest part of the vascular 3D printing literature refers to the preoperative simulation of AAA. Tangible 3D models allow vascular surgeons to study the unique anatomical structure or abnormalities of the aorta, in order to have a better insight of the best endovascular treatment modality (appropriate endografts, custom-made modification, chimney- or fenestrated endovascular repair) and the assessment of technical and clinical success [6].

Meess et al. applied 3D printing for preoperative guidance and surgical planning in an AAA treated with fenestrated endovascular aneurysm repair (FEVAR). The patient's specific 3D model served as a diagnostic tool and training "device" in a risk-free environment. Also, the phantom proved to be a useful tool in detecting possible periprocedural complications. Therefore, the model guided the authors to modify their surgical plan in order to avoid any complication, decrease the procedural time, and avoid unnecessary challenges during surgery. Moreover, the team had time to practice with the implanting device, leading to a reduction in radiation exposure of both patient and surgical staff, anesthesia, and contrast agent to the patient. 3D printing model has been shown to be more effective with respect to preoperational planning compared to the standard planning based on CTA diagnostic imaging alone [15]. Takao et al. reported on applied rapid prototyping in order to produce a model of hollow splenic artery aneurysm. The 3D model served as a simulation aid to endovascular treatment. An FDM-type desktop 3D printer and computed-tomography angiography data were used. While the thickness of the layer was 0.2 mm, thinner layers could be further produced using other 3D printing techniques, such as STL and inkjet printing. Nonetheless, the mean cross-sectional areas were slightly smaller than those of the original mask images, with a maximum difference of 0.33 cm^2, rendering a precise and accurate model [16].

Rapid prototyping can clearly help endograft planning when facing issues such as dealing with complex anatomical issues and CT imaging that hinder proper and thorough reconstructions and measurements. Likewise, Tam et al. reported on a patient who had an infrarenal aortic aneurysm of 6.6 cm with severe neck angulation of approximately 90°. Because of the hostile neck anatomy, the most suitable endograft choice and the proper mode of intraoperative deployment of the device was obscure. Consequently, the CT data were segmented, processed, and converted into a stereolithographic format representing the lumen as a 3D volume, from which a full-sized replica was printed within 24 h. Careful inspection of the 3D aneurysm model revealed an adequate infrarenal sealing zone and led to the optimal choice of an endograft. Accordingly, the authors suggested that the rapid prototype can assist the surgical team not only in AAA cases of angulated neck anatomy, but also in cases of short or conical neck [17].

Another complex neck anatomy of infrarenal AAA was successfully managed with the use of 3D printed models. In this case, the infrarenal AAA had a severely angled (approximately 90°) and short neck. The greatest difficulty in such cases is to predict the possible changes in neck shape, after the deployment of a stent, since this could lead to deployment outside or improper deployment of the endograft leading to inadvertent coverage of renal ostia or improper sealing. Hence, it is crucial to find a way to predict any potential outcome after the stent deployment. Since this cannot be easily done with the available conservative imaging methods, surgeons can draw useful information by means of creating a 3D printed model. The model helped the team in surgical planning and the selection of the appropriate approach, thus minimizing the intervention time [18].

3D printing has been also implicated in decision making and treatment of challenging thoracic aortic aneurysms (TAA) and dissections. In such cases, the main problem focuses on prediction of the change of the aortic arch angle after stent deployment, which could possibly result in the formation of a new lesion or even cause reverse extension. Thus, production of 3D models aids in better decision making and facilitates the optimal choice of endograft. In addition, surgical simulation enables vascular surgeons to avoid any difficulties in the use of guidewires and changes their approach in order to ensure the technical success of surgery [18].

Knox et al. reported on three patients with arterial abnormalities, those being high-grade stenosis of the right common artery bifurcation, basilar tip aneurysm, and abdominal aortic aneurysm. The created 3D models were accurate enough to reproduce flow dynamics of the altered anatomy. Obviously, the unique advantage of 3D printing is that the surgeon can have a preoperative hands-on experience with the pathology he plans to interfere with. As one rotates the reconstructed 3D model in every direction and experiments with it, one develops a haptic intuition concerning the best surgical approach [19]. Hence, as noted by Petzold et al., the 3D model introduces a new kind of interaction called **"touch to comprehend."**

A traverse arch hypoplasia model has also been presented. The model was very accurate with respect to magnetic resonance- and X-ray angiographic images with only a minor deviation of 0.36 ± 0.45 mm. One can easily appreciate this accuracy since catheter interventions, especially in children, rely strongly on the proper sizing of stents and balloons, with quite narrow variations. Hence, 3D models have been shown to be useful in terms of determining the size of the balloon, the stent length, and optimal position. Furthermore, modification and advances allow mimicking expansion of the vessel wall during balloon inflation [9]. More specifically, 3D models are not only used for preoperative simulation, but also during the operation as a guide for the specialists, even more in combination with robotic surgery [20]. The models play a major role in testing catheters and wires in a full-scale anatomically accurate vascular model, as the equipment performance can be evaluated in a controlled environment in the patient's unique anatomy [21].

Bioprinting

The use of 3D printing in medicine is being developed through the last years. In vascular surgery, rapid prototyping is getting involved in creating vascular tissue customized for each patient, created with the use of a 3D printer. Bioprinting efforts have enabled the fabrication of biologically functional blood vessels [22,23].

Lee et al. (2014) suggested a method for constructing endothelialized fluidic channels (lumen size of ~ 1 mm), the formation of adjacent capillary network with consequent generation of multiscale vascular network by connecting 1-mm-scale vessels with microvasculatures [24]. 3D bioprinting technique is combined either with the biological self-assembling of endothelial cells in scaffolds, gelatin methacrylate (GelMA), hydrogel using UV photocrosslinking [25], or a combination of electrospinning and 3D bioprinting system [26]. According to in vitro experiments, a 3D printed network can provide adequate levels of oxygen and support the viability of differentiating human mesenchymal stem cells under specific circumstances and perfusion bioreactors [27]. There has also been description of techniques for constructed triple-layer 3D vascular grafts [28].

Future use of such 3D printed vascular networks in humans is promising, as Melchiorri et al. have shown that noncellular 3D printed propylene fumarate vessels had a 6-month patency and functionality in mice after transplantation in their venous system [29]. Latest in vivo experiments presented implantation of 3D printed vascular networks for angiogenesis. The experimental products were implanted in mice with limb ischemia. The perfusion distally at the feet progressively increased, with a nonischemic limb at 5 days postoperatively [30].

Training and education

One of the most promising aspects of 3D printing is teaching anatomy to medical students. O'Reilly et al. produced a 3D model of lower limp, in order to assist medical students learn lower limp anatomy, as well as a femoral artery/vein model to train them in femoral vessel access. Even though, cadaveric dissection is the main way to learn anatomy for centuries, the efficiency of 3D printing in producing accurate anatomical models is drawing attention concerning the teaching progress. It is worth mentioning that the 3D model of the leg was considered as useful as the cadaveric-based teaching. Moreover, the printed reconstruction of femoral vessels has proven beneficial in training students to surgically access these vessels [31].

Medical prototypes are used through the training of junior doctors and interns of vascular surgery. It is recognized that endovascular procedures demand high level of accuracy and abilities that have always been taught entirely through a training-model involving patients exclusively. Not long-ago, virtual simulation (VR) gained importance and managed to be validated for educational reasons [32]. An alternative method for training in endovascular surgery is practicing on cadaveric specimens, despite the fact that this practice requires financial resources and is, in many situations, nonpractical [33].

The traditional mantra of "see one, do one, teach one" is now being replaced by "see one, sim many, do one." Considering that both methods, VR and cadaveric simulation, are highly expensive and require an ongoing technical support, a different approach should be followed which should be simple, inexpensive, and technically nondemanding in order to achieve improvement in endovascular training and pave the way to an extensive use of simulation in surgical training [34]. In the study of Mafeld et al., a 3D printed endovascular simulation was put into the test by 96 physicians. They answered 12 questions evaluating the use and feasibility of 3D printed anatomically accurate aortic model for training purposes. According to the study, most of the physicians agreed that 3D models were realistic compared to live patients and VR, in the fields of vascular access, guidewire- and catheter manipulation, and vessel catheterization. Moreover, most physicians agreed that 3D printed model was a useful tool for basic training and improved their handing skills. There was also wide agreement regarding the importance of its future use. 3D printed modeling is considered a valuable learning tool, accompanied by strong recommendations for further involvement by teaching hospitals [35].

Postoperative studies and academic purposes

Medical rapid prototyping offers a great opportunity for studies concerning computational fluid dynamics and mechanisms of vascular pathologies.

Studying flow dynamics in vascular prototypes starts with the examination of geometric parameters, including the branching angle, maximum curvature at the apex, and volume of the branch. Han et al. have already shown that large joining angles make no difference to the hemodynamic behavior, as most capillary junctions have large joining angles [36]. There have been several methods described in order to manage the distal arterial flow resistance and pressure, thus creating physiologically and geometrically accurate models that can be also used for simulations of image-guided interventional procedures with new devices, but also for physiological simulations [37]. Canstein et al. since 2008 have shown that in vitro model systems, such as 3D printed vascular prototypes, could successfully be used to analyze local and global flow dynamics in a realistic one-to-one replica of normal in vivo thoracic aortic anatomy [38]. Moreover, Ahmadian et al. demonstrate the feasibility of combining in vivo MRI and 3D printing for the comprehensive evaluation of aortic abnormalities like dissection, but also enables in vitro simulation of interventions like graft repair on aortic flow characteristics, opening new horizons in procedural planning [39].

At an experimental level, a method called "Ring Stacking Method" by Pinnock et al. was described as a way to create artificial arteries of various dimensions and lengths, using 3D printed guides. With this method, variable size rings of vascular smooth muscle cells can be created using guides of center posts to control lumen diameter and outer shells to dictate vessel wall thickness. These tissue rings are then stacked to create a tubular construct, mimicking the natural form of a blood vessel [40].

Costa et al. in 2017 demonstrated methods for manufacturing microfluidic cell culture models in vitro, by combining CTA data and 3D printing, developing a new approach which precisely mimics the architectures found in both healthy and stenotic arteries. With this approach, thrombosis can be recapitulated in 3D vessel geometries in a way that is not possible in microfluidic chips fabricated with typical 2D wafer-based soft lithography, or even in microfluidic chips produced with acrylic fibers or by advanced biofabrication methods [41].

Conclusion

As it can be clearly seen in this chapter, 3D printing is a technology with multiple applications in both vascular and endovascular surgery, in terms of educating medical students, residents, and fellows, as well as testing the potential graft preoperatively and being able to plan the operation. The bottom line is that it can help vascular surgeons increase the safety and quality of their work, something which will directly benefit our patients.

References

[1] Shi D, Liu K, Zhang X, et al. Applications of three-dimensional printing technology in the cardiovascular field. Intern Emerg Med 2015;10(7):769−80.

[2] Singare S, Liu Y, Li D, et al. Individually prefabricated prosthesis for maxilla reconstuction. J Prosthodont 2008;17(2):135−40.

[3] Jacobs S, Grunert R, Mohr FW, et al. 3D-Imaging of cardiac structures using 3D heart models for planning in heart surgery: a preliminary study. Interact Cardiovasc Thorac Surg 2008;7(1):6−9.

[4] Subburaj K, Nair C, Rajesh S, et al. Rapid development of auricular prosthesis using CAD and rapid prototyping technologies. Int J Oral Maxillofac Surg 2007;36(10): 938−43.

[5] Youssef RF, Spradling K, Yoon R, et al. Applications of three-dimensional printing technology in urological practice. BJU Int 2015;116(5):697−702.

[6] Bangeas P, Voulalas G, Ktenidis K. Rapid prototyping in aortic surgery. Interact Cardiovasc Thorac Surg 2016;22(4):513−4.

[7] Ho D, Squelch A, Sun Z. Modelling of aortic aneurysm and aortic dissection through 3D printing. J Med Radiat Sci 2017;64(1):10−7.

[8] Chick JFB, Reddy SN, Yu AC, et al. Three-dimensional printing facilitates successful endovascular closure of a type II abernethy malformation using an amplatzer atrial septal occluder device. Ann Vasc Surg 2017;43. 311 e315−311 e323.

[9] Valverde I, Gomez G, Coserria JF, et al. 3D printed models for planning endovascular stenting in transverse aortic arch hypoplasia. Cathet Cardiovasc Interv 2015;85(6): 1006−12.

[10] Maragiannis D, Jackson MS, Igo SR, et al. Replicating patient-specific severe aortic valve stenosis with functional 3D modeling. Circ Cardiovasc Imag 2015;8(10): e003626.

[11] Maragiannis D, Jackson MS, Igo SR, et al. Functional 3D printed patient-specific modeling of severe aortic stenosis. J Am Coll Cardiol 2014;64(10):1066−8.

[12] Schievano S, Migliavacca F, Coats L, et al. Percutaneous pulmonary valve implantation based on rapid prototyping of right ventricular outflow tract and pulmonary trunk from MR data. Radiology 2007;242(2):490−7.

[13] Milosavljevic S, Milburn PD, Knox BW. The influence of occupation on lumbar sagittal motion and posture. Ergonomics 2005;48(6):657−67.

[14] Takao H, Amemiya S, Shibata E, et al. Three-dimensional printing of hollow portal vein stenosis models: a feasibility study. J Vasc Interv Radiol 2016;27(11):1755−8.

[15] Meess KM, Izzo RL, Dryjski ML, et al. 3D printed abdominal aortic aneurysm phantom for image guided surgical planning with a patient specific fenestrated endovascular graft system. Proc SPIE-Int Soc Opt Eng 2017:10138.

[16] Takao H, Amemiya S, Shibata E, et al. 3D printing of preoperative simulation models of a splenic artery aneurysm: precision and accuracy. Acad Radiol 2017;24(5):650−3.

[17] Tam MD, Laycock SD, Brown JR, et al. 3D printing of an aortic aneurysm to facilitate decision making and device selection for endovascular aneurysm repair in complex neck anatomy. J Endovasc Ther 2013;20(6):863−7.

[18] Yuan D, Luo H, Yang H, et al. Precise treatment of aortic aneurysm by three-dimensional printing and simulation before endovascular intervention. Sci Rep 2017; 7(1):795.

[19] Knox K, Kerber CW, Singel SA, et al. Stereolithographic vascular replicas from CT scans: choosing treatment strategies, teaching, and research from live patient scan data. AJNR Am J Neuroradiol 2005;26(6):1428−31.

[20] Salloum C, Lim C, Fuentes L, et al. Fusion of information from 3D printing and surgical robot: an innovative minimally technique illustrated by the resection of a large celiac trunk aneurysm. World J Surg 2016;40(1):245−7.

[21] Itagaki MW. Using 3D printed models for planning and guidance during endovascular intervention: a technical advance. Diagn Interv Radiol 2015;21(4):338−41.

[22] Yu Y, Zhang Y, Martin JA, et al. Evaluation of cell viability and functionality in vessel-like bioprintable cell-laden tubular channels. J Biomech Eng 2013;135(9):91011.

[23] Skardal A, Zhang J, Prestwich GD. Bioprinting vessel-like constructs using hyaluronan hydrogels crosslinked with tetrahedral polyethylene glycol tetracrylates. Biomaterials 2010;31(24):6173−81.

[24] Lee VK, Lanzi AM, Haygan N, et al. Generation of multi-scale vascular network system within 3D hydrogel using 3D bio-printing technology. Cell Mol Bioeng 2014;7(3): 460−72.

[25] Yang L, Shridhar SV, Gerwitz M, et al. An in vitro vascular chip using 3D printing-enabled hydrogel casting. Biofabrication 2016;8(3):035015.

[26] Lee SJ, Heo DN, Park JS, et al. Characterization and preparation of bio-tubular scaffolds for fabricating artificial vascular grafts by combining electrospinning and a 3D printing system. Phys Chem Chem Phys 2015;17(5):2996−9.

[27] Ball O, Nguyen BB, Placone JK, et al. 3D printed vascular networks enhance viability in high-volume perfusion bioreactor. Ann Biomed Eng 2016;44(12):3435−45.

[28] Huang R, Gao X, Wang J, et al. Triple-layer vascular grafts fabricated by combined E-Jet 3D printing and electrospinning. Ann Biomed Eng 2018;46(9):1254−66.

[29] Melchiorri AJ, Hibino N, Best CA, et al. 3D-Printed biodegradable polymeric vascular grafts. Adv Healthc Mater 2016;5(3):319−25.

[30] Mirabella T, MacArthur JW, Cheng D, et al. 3D-printed vascular networks direct therapeutic angiogenesis in ischaemia. Nat Biomed Eng 2017;1.

[31] O'Reilly MK, Reese S, Herlihy T, et al. Fabrication and assessment of 3D printed anatomical models of the lower limb for anatomical teaching and femoral vessel access training in medicine. Anat Sci Educ 2016;9(1):71−9.

[32] Rudarakanchana N, Van Herzeele I, Desender L, et al. Virtual reality simulation for the optimization of endovascular procedures: current perspectives. Vasc Health Risk Manag 2015;11:195−202.

[33] Chevallier C, Willaert W, Kawa E, et al. Postmortem circulation: a new model for testing endovascular devices and training clinicians in their use. Clin Anat 2014; 27(4):556−62.

[34] Nelson K, Bagnall A, Nesbitt C, et al. Developing cross-specialty endovascular simulation training. Clin Teach 2014;11(6):411−5.

[35] Mafeld S, Nesbitt C, McCaslin J, et al. Three-dimensional (3D) printed endovascular simulation models: a feasibility study. Ann Transl Med 2017;5(3):42.

[36] Han X, Bibb R, Harris R. Engineering design of artificial vascular junctions for 3D printing. Biofabrication 2016;8(2):025018.

[37] Sommer K, Izzo RL, Shepard L, et al. Design optimization for accurate flow simulations in 3D printed vascular phantoms derived from computed tomography angiography. Proc SPIE-Int Soc Opt Eng 2017:10138.

[38] Canstein C, Cachot P, Faust A, et al. 3D MR flow analysis in realistic rapid-prototyping model systems of the thoracic aorta: comparison with in vivo data and computational fluid dynamics in identical vessel geometries. Magn Reson Med 2008;59(3):535–46.

[39] Rouzbeh RA, A PB, Alessandro MS, Jeremy DC, James CC, Patrick MMC, Malaisrie SC, Barker AJ, Markl M. Comprehensive evaluation of aortic disease by in-vivo 4D flow MRI and 3D printing of patient-specific models: a feasibility study. J Cardiovasc Magn Reson 2016;18(Suppl. 1):365.

[40] Pinnock CB, Xu Z, Lam MT. Scaling of engineered vascular grafts using 3D printed guides and the ring stacking method. J Vis Exp 2017;121.

[41] Costa PF, Albers HJ, Linssen JEA, et al. Mimicking arterial thrombosis in a 3D-printed microfluidic in vitro vascular model based on computed tomography angiography data. Lab Chip 2017;17(16):2785–92.

3D printing in orthopedic surgery

Anastasios-Nektarios Tzavellas, MD, MSc [1,2,3],
Eustathios Kenanidis, MD, PhD, MSc [1,2], **Michael Potoupnis, MD, PhD** [1,2],
Eleftherios Tsiridis, MD, MSc, PhD, FACS, FRCS [1,2]

[1]*Academic Orthopaedic Department, Papageorgiou General Hospital, Aristotle University Medical School, Thessaloniki, Greece;* [2]*Center of Orthopaedic and Regenerative Medicine (C.O. RE.) - Center for Interdisciplinary Research and Innovation — Aristotle University Thessaloniki (C. I.R.I.-AU.Th), Balkan Center, Buildings A & B, Thessaloniki, Greece;* [3]*Orthopaedic Surgeon, 2nd Department of Orthopaedic and Trauma Surgery, 424 Military General Hospital, Thessaloniki, Greece*

Introduction

The advancements in medical imaging, including improvements on hardware and software of computed tomography (CT) and magnetic resonance imaging (MRI), have provided an easier, more reliable, and more accurate diagnosis and treatment planning. Although three-dimensional (3D) reconstruction images offer good visualization of the anatomic structures, they do not produce the prehension of a physical model.

3D printing is an emerging technology that uses an appropriate computer software in order to build objects by data. Since its first application in medicine, the usage of 3D printing has firmly gained attention and subscribers, especially among surgical specialties [1]. During the last 5 years, an increasing trend in research and publications over applications of 3D printing in Orthopedic Surgery has been noticed [2]. This trend was supported by technological developments of 3D printers, the lowering of their cost, and the handling of new materials. Various powder-like or gel-like materials are described to have been utilized, such as plastics, metals, polymers, ceramics, as well as biological materials (Table 10.1).

Anatomic models
Operative planning

Traditional preoperative planning relies on plain X-rays and 2D or 3D CT images. There have been significant advances in image processing technologies; however, 3D anatomy is still viewed as a flat image. 3D printers process these data and build a full-scale physical 3D model. These models provide a tactile impression and a better understanding of the patients' normal and pathological anatomy and

3D Printing: Applications in Medicine and Surgery. https://doi.org/10.1016/B978-0-323-66164-5.00010-6

Table 10.1 Materials used commonly for 3D printing applications in Orthopedics.

Sintered powder metal	Thermoplastic polymers (polypropylene, polyether ether ketone, polyether ketone)
Metals (stainless steel, nitinol, titanium)	Polycaprolactone (PCL)
Bone-like (CT-bone)	Bioceramics (hydroxyapatite, tricalcium phosphate [TCP], calcium phosphate, silica, bioglass, zinc oxide)
Plastics (polyethylene acetate)	Gelatin and collagen
Polyurethane	Poly-L-lactic acid (PLLA)
Styrene	Bioinks

pathophysiology. Patient-specific anatomical characteristics and variations are easily visualized. Review of 3D-printed models preoperatively can help surgeons to select the appropriate approach and to forerun potential difficulties or the need for special equipment [3—6].

Orthopedic trauma is a suitable field for application of 3D-printed models, especially when regions with complex anatomy are involved (i.e., acetabular or intra-articular fractures). Hurson et al. and Bagaria et al. proved that these models assisted surgeons to meliorate the understanding of individual anatomy and complex acetabular fracture patterns [7,8]. Since the first utilization of 3D printing in trauma patients, it has proliferated to almost all anatomic areas [5] (Table 10.2).

Providing a multiangle and multidirectional view, it increases reliability and accuracy of diagnosis and classification of the fractures. Surgeons can plan the maneuvers of reduction and fixation. Using the mirror imaging technique and the normal, uninjured side as a template, they can choose the positioning of the reduction clumps, select the appropriate plate and its optimal placement, measure its length, and pre-bend it in order to fit the anatomic region where it will be placed. The number of screws needed, their location and entry points, length, and trajectories can be determined a priori [5,9—11].In particular, 3D printing assistance is considerable when inexperienced surgeons face a complex fracture, while experienced ones find it less useful or even unnecessary when dealing with a simple fracture pattern [12]. 3D models can also be sterilized and brought into the operation room and used as references. Operations can be performed on the printed models at the doctor's desk, transforming virtual stimulation into realistic stimulation, and this "hands-on" approach is appreciated by many surgeons [5,11].

As a result, operation time, intraoperative blood loss, and overall fluoroscopies are reduced. Minimally invasive techniques can be used even at complex fractures as the accuracy of reduction and fixation is increased. Complications, such as iatrogenic nerve injuries, are decreased [5,6,9,10,12].

Table 10.2 Summary of 3D printing applications per area in Orthopedic trauma.

Anatomic region	Application
Upper limb	
Acromion	Model for plate precontouring, patient–surgeon communication
Clavicle	Model for preoperative planning, reduction techniques, MIPO, plate precontouring
Proximal humerus	Model for preoperative planning, simulating operation
Distal humerus, elbow	3D-printed plates, model for preoperative planning, patient–surgeon communication, patient-specific instruments
Distal radius	Model for preoperative planning, patient-specific instruments
Hand	Model for preoperative planning (thumb reconstruction, vascularized skin flaps and bone grafts)
Lower limb	
Acetabulum	Model for preoperative planning, plate precontouring, resident training, patient–surgeon communication, simulating operation, intraoperative reference, patient-specific instruments
Pelvis	Model for preoperative planning, simulating operation, 3D-printed drill guides
Distal femur	Model for preoperative planning, patient-specific instruments
Proximal tibia	Model for preoperative planning, patient–surgeon communication
ACL reconstruction	3D-printed tunnel guides for anatomical reconstruction
Pilon and malleoli fractures	Model for preoperative planning, templating, plate precontouring, patient–surgeon communication,
Talus, calcaneus, foot	Model for preoperative planning, templating, plate precontouring, patient–surgeon communication, 3D-printed plates
Spine	
Fracture-dislocations	Model for preoperative planning, templates for pedicles screws

Spine surgery is another field of Orthopedics where 3D printing has potentially a wide range of applications. 3D models are used in cases with spinal deformities (i.e., idiopathic scoliosis, kyphosis, meningomyelocele) and help the study of joint inclination, false articulations, and pedicle size. These models were utilized in the preoperative setting for the planning of curve correction and pedicle screw placement, resulting in a safer and more accurate operation [6,13,14].

Pediatric Orthopedic surgeons have used 3D models to manage foot deformities, Perthes or Blount disease. Osteotomies in either pediatric or adult patients can also be planned with the aid of such models. The surgeon can study the deformity, choose the ideal site for the osteotomy, and prepare the angle of correction in all planes providing him with confidence during operation [6].

Educational applications

The potential applications for the education of residents and junior surgeons have not been evaluated as thoroughly. There are numerous theoretical benefits. Surgical training in Orthopedics is mostly done in the operation theater or on cadavers. On the other hand, practicing on 3D-printed models offers to trainees a tangible, reproducible, and easy-to-understand format. It also provides trainers and seniors with a more accessible and safer way to communicate their knowledge and experience. Files can be saved, stored, or even shared among institutions. Patient-specific 3D models can be printed again and again on demand providing a collection of even rare and complex cases that can be used without any limitations for surgical practicing, equipping residents with familiarity and confidence before entering the operation theater [3,6,15–18].

Doctor–patient communication

3D-printed models can be critical during a discussion between an Orthopedic surgeon and a patient and can assist in the consent process. Patient education is a significant part of modern patient-centered healthcare systems. Showing the anatomic 3D model to the patients and their familiars will help them to better understand their pathology, as well as the operation that will take place and the risks that have to overcome, especially in complex trauma patients or with spine deformities [1,3,6,13,16,17].

Patient-specific implants and instruments

Advances in 3D printing technology have highlighted the fabrication of patient-specific implants. Joint arthroplasty and orthopedic oncology are mostly the fields of interest. Although custom-made, patient-specific knee implants are available for primary, noncomplex knee arthroplasty, such customized implants are better suitable for patients whose bone anatomy is outside the range of standard implants regarding implant size or disease-specific requirements. Patients with dwarfism, hip dysplasia, revision arthroplasty, and bone tumor resection are examples of such cases [3,4,6,11,17] (Table 10.3).

3D-printed implants can be provided with a porous surface similar to the conventional implants in order to facilitate osteointegration, minimize stress shielding and ensure long-term survival. They also can be manufactured by trabecular metals. Custom-made implants are accompanied with a set of individualized tools for replicating the planned bone cuts, custom-made trial implants, and drill guides to facilitate accurate placement of the prosthesis. Full-scale models for preoperative planning and intraoperative reference and guidance are provided too.

Table 10.3 Applications of 3D-printed, custom-made implants.

Medical condition	Problems solved—advantages
Dwarfism	Patients too small for conventional implants
Hip dysplasia	Acetabular dysplasia, proximal femur deformities due to past operations
Revision hip arthroplasty	Implant fits the defect site accurately, especially for significant defects as Paprosky type 3, improve osteointegration, trabecular implants
Spine deformities	Anterior and posterior intervertebral fusion cage implants, lowered rate of implant dislocation and subsidence, improved correction of deformity primary stabilization
Oncology	Implants fit the defect site, the existence of preplanned soft tissue attachment sites, used at osteosarcomas, pelvic chondrosarcomas, spine tumors, tumors of clavicle, scapula, calcaneus

Despite the patient-specific aid and instrumentation, malpositioning of such implants is not rare. On the contrary, accurate placement is still considered challenging, as intraoperative flexibility is absent. Custom-made implants require time to be designed and manufactured, while the cost is significantly higher than the traditional ones. If long-term survival and excellent outcomes were granted, 3D printing would be cost-effective as revision arthroplasty due to conventional implant earlier loosening would be costly. Unfortunately, this benefit has yet to be proven. There were not even significantly favorable short-term outcomes that could justify 3D-printed, custom-made implants for primary arthroplasty.

Patient-specific instruments (PSIs) are used trying to efficiently and accurately repeat the operative plan. In Orthopedics, this mainly involves a saw and drill guide for working in a preplanned direction. 3D printing is utilized in creating PSIs by either printing directly the instrument or printing a real-size anatomic model that will be the template for conventionally fabricating the final instrument. Such 3D-printed PSIs have been reported in pedicle screw insertion for spinal surgery, internal fixation of acetabular fractures, templates for osteotomies to correct bone deformities or malunion of fractures, and saw guides used in arthroplasty [17]. The most important limitation of PSIs is their potential incorrect positioning and the inability to realize it intraoperatively. Improvements in imaging technology and the accuracy of printed models will motivate PSI technology.

Casts and orthotics

Plaster or fiberglass casts and splints are applied for the treatment of most fracture patients. They can be used either after closed reduction as a permanent, conservative treatment or after an operation. These casts are generated by the surface anatomy of the injured limbs. Patients suffer mechanical pressure during molding and application procedure while lack of reproducibility is an additional disadvantage. Traditional casts create discomfort due to weight, poor ventilation, and skin problems [19−21]. A cast that is not well-set leads to abnormally applied forces on the injured limb. As a result, the reduction can be lost; the fracture can be malunited, and local pressure sores can develop.

These features led to an interest in 3D printing, and the need for the development of applications for rehabilitation tools was created. Techniques of 3D printing patient-specific casts for the treatment of distal radius fractures both in adults and children are well described [19,20]. Initial research on simple fractures shows the noninferiority of such casts compared to the traditional ones. Fracture healing, complication rates, and functionality after the removal of the cast were comparable between two groups in all studies [19−23]. Nevertheless, patients expressed a preference for the 3D-printed casts, as the pressure-related complications were diminished and the super-lightweight and well-ventilated design abridged intervention in patients' daily activities increasing their satisfaction. On the other hand, the need for the initial application of a plaster cast cannot still be eliminated. After closed reduction, primary stabilization with a traditional cast is necessary in order to proceed to the scanning technique for the manufacturing of the 3D-printed cast. Increased cost and time required to print a patient-specific cast are issues that should be solved [19−23].

Orthotics are externally worn medical devices used to modify the structural and functional characteristics of the neuromuscular and skeletal system. Ankle-foot orthotics (AFO) are used to support the lower leg, to manage deformities and imbalance. They are traditionally applied to patients with cerebral palsy, stroke, head injuries, multiple sclerosis, and clubfoot. AFOs are made using thermoplastic vacuum forming over a positive model. This is a labor-assuming and time-consuming technique with several design constraints. 3D printing technology offers design freedom and manufacture of patient-specific AFOs with theoretically optimized biomechanics, improved functionality, better fit, and aesthetics [24,25]. However, 3D-printed AFOs seem to be still under research and experimental perusal, and their clinical application lacks firm verification [25].

Great enthusiasm has been generated over the last years for the development and manufacture of 3D-printed upper limb prosthesis. A fast quest on the web will emerge several products, such as Robohand, Andrianesis' hand, Cyborg beast, IVI-ANA. 3D-printed prosthesis offers a cheaper alternative to those who cannot afford the commercial ones. As mentioned above, 3D printing offers design freedom. The prosthesis can be personalized, rapidly constructed, while improvements can fit each patient's needs. On the other hand, there are significant limitations in complexity, size, and materials that can be used [26].

Tissue engineering

Bone tissue engineering is a multidisciplinary field of science aiming to create a structure to regenerate new bone or cartilage. A structural scaffold is provided for cell attachment and proliferation, which lead to bone or cartilage formation. 3D printing has recently attracted attention for the research on the development of such scaffolds.

CT or MRI depicts a patient's defect, and its parameters are digitized and used in order to print a scaffold that exactly matches the initial defect. 3D printing technology has the advantage of fabricating patient-specific scaffolds with even complex shape and anatomy, which is quite hard to achieve with conventional scaffold fabrication techniques [17,27–29]. 3D-printed scaffolds are also manufactured faster and more cost-effectively than traditional methods.

Mechanical properties and structural parameters, such as porosity, pore size, and interconnectivity, can be precisely defined. Biomaterials used to offer that advantage of biocompatibility, nontoxicity, and biodegradability [30,31]. New bioceramics can be utilized, while the combination of natural and ceramic materials or different ceramics is now possible (Table 10.1) [28–30]. Loading scaffold with cells, drugs, and bioactive molecules can offer the advantage of guiding the cell microenvironment and multipotency to differentiation to specific tissue regeneration [27,32].

Future perspectives

3D printing technologies have the potential of causing a revolution in Orthopedic Surgery. The so enviable individualized medicine seems closer to becoming a reality. The consolidation, though, in everyday clinical and academic practice depends on whether future advances will be able to outflank the stated disadvantages. The lowering of their cost makes 3D printers more accessible. Printing speed and accuracy have been increased, and printers are easier to handle.

Mechanical properties of 3D-printed objects should be ameliorated. Materials used in 3D printing applications in Orthopedics are metals, ceramics, and polymers. Objects fabricated by them using 3D printing technology are still inferior to the traditional ones. Safety of such technology, guidelines, and regulations controlling applications are more than necessary.

Biological 3D printing remains a significant challenge. Restoring and emulating the bone complex microenvironment and the macroscopic functionality and properties are still an illusion. Current applications consist of printing scaffold and loading it with cells and growth factors. Bioink technology is nowadays evolving.

Educational applications and modeling for preoperative planning are possible implementations. Long-term follow-up and high-quality clinical studies are necessary to reveal the pragmatic impact of this technology in Orthopedic Surgery.

References

[1] Martelli N, Serrano C, van den Brink H, Pineau J, Prognon P, Borget I, et al. Advantages and disadvantages of 3-dimensional printing in surgery: a systematic review. Surgery 2016;159(6):1485—500.

[2] Vaishya R, Patralekh MK, Vaish A, Agarwal AK, Vijay V. Publication trends and knowledge mapping in 3D printing in orthopaedics. Materials 2018;9(3):194—201.

[3] Aimar A, Palermo A, Innocenti B. The role of 3D printing in medical applications: a state of the art. J Healthc Eng 2019;2019:5340616.

[4] Eltorai AE, Nguyen E, Daniels AH. Three-dimensional printing in orthopedic surgery. Orthopedics 2015;38(11):684—7.

[5] Lal H, Patralekh MK. 3D printing and its applications in orthopaedic trauma: a technological marvel. J Clin Orthop Trauma 2018;9(3):260—8.

[6] Mulford JS, Babazadeh S, Mackay N. Three-dimensional printing in orthopaedic surgery: review of current and future applications. ANZ J Surg 2016;86(9):648—53.

[7] Bagaria V, Deshpande S, Rasalkar DD, Kuthe A, Paunipagar BK. Use of rapid prototyping and three-dimensional reconstruction modeling in the management of complex fractures. Eur J Radiol 2011;80(3):814—20.

[8] Hurson C, Tansey A, O'Donnchadha B, Nicholson P, Rice J, McElwain J. Rapid prototyping in the assessment, classification and preoperative planning of acetabular fractures. Injury 2007;38(10):1158—62.

[9] Liu ZJ, Jia J, Zhang YG, Tian W, Jin X, Hu YC. Internal fixation of complicated acetabular fractures directed by preoperative surgery with 3D printing models. Orthop Surg 2017;9(2):257—60.

[10] Wan L, Zhang X, Zhang S, Li K, Cao P, Li J, et al. Clinical feasibility and application value of computer virtual reduction combined with 3D printing technique in complex acetabular fractures. Exp Ther Med 2019;17(5):3630—6.

[11] Wong TM, Jin J, Lau TW, Fang C, Yan CH, Yeung K, et al. The use of three-dimensional printing technology in orthopaedic surgery. J Orthop Surg 2017;25(1). 2309499016684077.

[12] Kang HJ, Kim BS, Kim SM, Kim YM, Kim HN, Park JY, et al. Can preoperative 3D printing change surgeon's operative plan for distal tibia fracture? BioMed Res Int 2019;2019:7059413.

[13] Cho W, Job AV, Chen J, Baek JH. A review of current clinical applications of three-dimensional printing in spine surgery. Asian Spine J 2018;12(1):171—7.

[14] Garg B, Gupta M, Singh M, Kalyanasundaram D. Outcome and safety analysis of 3D-printed patient-specific pedicle screw jigs for complex spinal deformities: a comparative study. Spine J 2019;19(1):56—64.

[15] Michalski MH, Ross JS. The shape of things to come: 3D printing in medicine. JAMA 2014;312(21):2213—4.

[16] Niikura T, Sugimoto M, Lee SY, Sakai Y, Nishida K, Kuroda R, et al. Tactile surgical navigation system for complex acetabular fracture surgery. Orthopedics 2014;37(4): 237—42.

[17] Wong KC. 3D-printed patient-specific applications in orthopedics. Orthop Res Rev 2016;8:57—66.

[18] Manganaro MS, Morag Y, Weadock WJ, Yablon CM, Gaetke-Udager K, Stein EB. Creating three-dimensional printed models of acetabular fractures for use as educational tools. Radiographics 2017;37(3):871−80.

[19] Chen YJ, Lin H, Zhang X, Huang W, Shi L, Wang D. Application of 3D-printed and patient-specific cast for the treatment of distal radius fractures: initial experience. 3D Print Med 2017;3(1):11.

[20] Guida P, Casaburi A, Busiello T, Lamberti D, Sorrentino A, Iuppariello L, et al. An alternative to plaster cast treatment in a pediatric trauma center using the CAD/CAM technology to manufacture customized three-dimensional-printed orthoses in a totally hospital context: a feasibility study. J Pediatr Orthop B 2019;28(3):248−55.

[21] Lin H, Shi L, Wang D. A rapid and intelligent designing technique for patient-specific and 3D-printed orthopedic cast. 3D Print Med 2015;2(1):4.

[22] Graham J, Wang M, Frizzell K, Watkins C, Beredjiklian P, Rivlin M. Conventional vs 3-dimensional printed cast wear comfort. New York, NY): Hand; 2018. 1558944718795291.

[23] Hoogervorst P, Knox R, Tanaka K, Working ZM, El Naga AN, Herfat S, et al. A biomechanical comparison of fiberglass casts and 3-dimensional-printed, open-latticed, ventilated casts. New York, NY: Hand; 2019. 1558944719831341.

[24] Wojciechowski E, Chang AY, Balassone D, Ford J, Cheng TL, Little D, et al. Feasibility of designing, manufacturing and delivering 3D printed ankle-foot orthoses: a systematic review. J Foot Ankle Res 2019;12:11.

[25] Xu R, Wang Z, Ma T, Ren Z, Jin H. Effect of 3D printing individualized ankle-foot orthosis on plantar biomechanics and pain in patients with plantar fasciitis: a randomized controlled trial. Med Sci Monit 2019;25:1392−400.

[26] Ten Kate J, Smit G, Breedveld P. 3D-printed upper limb prostheses: a review. Disabil Rehabil Assist Technol 2017;12(3):300−14.

[27] Marques CF, Diogo GS, Pina S, Oliveira JM, Silva TH, Reis RL. Collagen-based bio-inks for hard tissue engineering applications: a comprehensive review. J Tissue Eng Regenerat Med 2019;30(3):32.

[28] Midha S, Dalela M, Sybil D, Patra P, Mohanty S. Advances in three-dimensional bio-printing of bone: progress and challenges. J Tissue Eng Regen Med 2019;13(6):925−45.

[29] Wen Y, Xun S, Haoye M, Baichuan S, Peng C, Xuejian L, et al. 3D printed porous ceramic scaffolds for bone tissue engineering: a review. Biomater Sci 2017;5(9):1690−8.

[30] Moreno Madrid AP, Vrech SM, Sanchez MA, Rodriguez AP. Advances in additive manufacturing for bone tissue engineering scaffolds. Materials Sci Eng C Mater Biol Appl 2019;100:631−44.

[31] Theodoridis K, Aggelidou E, Vavilis T, Manthou ME, Tsimponis A, Demiri EC, et al. Hyaline cartilage next generation implants from adipose-tissue-derived mesenchymal stem cells: comparative study on 3D-printed polycaprolactone scaffold patterns. J Tissue Eng Regenerat Med 2019;13(2):342−55.

[32] Klontzas ME, Kenanidis EI, Heliotis M, Tsiridis E, Mantalaris A. Bone and cartilage regeneration with the use of umbilical cord mesenchymal stem cells. Expert Opin Biol Ther 2015;15(11):1541−52. https://doi.org/10.1517/14712598.2015.1068755. Epub 2015 Jul 15.

The role of 3D printing in ENT surgery

Marios Stavrakas, Petros D. Karkos, Jannis Constantinidis
ENT Department, Aristotle University of Thessaloniki, AHEPA Hospital, Thessaloniki, Greece

Introduction

Three-dimensional (3D) printing is a rapidly growing technology, with numerous applications in Otolaryngology and Head and Neck Surgery. Since its conception in the 1980s, 3D printing—also known as rapid prototyping, solid-freeform technology or additive manufacturing—technology and 3D printing equipment have improved and are less expensive; the expertise is more widespread, and therefore, it has been available in many parts of the world for medical use in several fields [1,2].

The concept of three-dimensional printing was introduced by C. Hull in 1986, and it was initially defined as an "apparatus for production of three-dimensional objects by stereolithography" [3,4]. As it is known, rapid prototyping involved the construction of three-dimensional models by gradually layering material [5]. The exact technology of 3D printing is still evolving and nowadays the ASTM International Committee F42 has described seven subcategories of 3D printing methodology, as shown in Table 11.1 [6]. All of them have their basis on the original principle of the .STL format (Standard Triangulation Language) which was developed by C. Hull in the 1980s and practically makes it possible to convert the surface of a three-dimensional object to triangles. There are several ways to obtain a .STL file format, such as DICOM data (digital imaging and communication in medicine) from CT or MRI scans, CAD (computer-aided design) software, or by scanning the actual object with an appropriate scanning device [3].

Apart from the subcategory classification in Table 11.1, it is worth mentioning the available technologies and the materials used, aiming to give an impression of the potential medical applications (Table 11.2). More detailed technical specifications and advantages/disadvantages are outside the scope of this chapter and therefore not analyzed in depth.

Applications in otolaryngology

Several articles can be found in the literature on the applications of 3D printing in Otolaryngology. These can be categorized according to the relevant subspecialty (Otology, Rhinology, Pediatric Otolaryngology, Head and Neck Surgery/Laryngology) but also according to the proposed application. Thus, the 3D-printed models

3D Printing: Applications in Medicine and Surgery. https://doi.org/10.1016/B978-0-323-66164-5.00011-8

Table 11.1 ASTM classification of 3D printing technologies [3,6].

Method	Brief description
I. Vat photopolymerization	A container gets filled with photopolymeric resin, which eventually gets hardened by a UV light source.
II. Material jetting	Material (photopolymeric resin) is dropped through small diameter nozzles and hardened by UV lamp.
III. Binder jetting	Powder base material spread in even layers and binder is used to "glue" the particles together to form the programmed 3D shape.
IV. Material extrusion	Thermoplastic filament that gets printed through a heating chamber, then moulded and solidified.
V. Power bed fusion	A high-power laser source fuses small particle of the selected material by scanning the cross- sections generated by the 3D modeling program on the surface of a power bed.
VI. Sheet lamination	Sheets of material are bound together through external force.
VII. Direct energy deposition	Creates 3D parts by melting material (usually metal) as it is being deposited.

Table 11.2 Examples of materials used in different 3D printing methods [1,39].

Method	Materials
1. Stereolithography	Photo-curable polymers, liquid resin
2. Fused deposition modeling	Structural and biopolymers, ceramic polymers or metal-polymer composites, solid thermoplastic filaments
3. Selective laser sintering	Powder materials (polymers, metals, ceramics)
4. 3D plotting	Polymers and ceramics (including polycaprolactone, hydroxyapatite, polylactic acid/polyethylene glycol)
5. Laser-assisted bioprinting	Hydroxyapatite, zirconia, HA/MG63, human osteoprogenitor cells, and human umbilical vein endothelial cells
6. Robotic-assisted deposition	Polycaprolactone, hydroxyapatite, bioactive glass, ceramics, ceramic-polymer composites

can be used in perioperative planning, patient education, surgical training, grafting, prosthetics, and reconstruction. A recent systematic review by Canzi et al. (2018) looked at 121 studies, with the majority of them focusing on perioperative planning and surgical training. It is also worth mentioning that this study demonstrated that most of the Head and Neck studies were relevant to preoperative planning, while ontological studies focused mainly on surgical training in terms of temporal bone

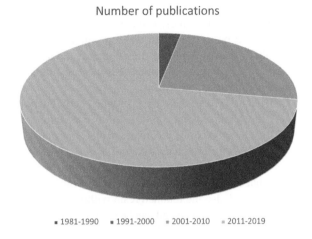

Number of publications

■ 1981-1990   ■ 1991-2000   ■ 2001-2010   ■ 2011-2019

FIGURE 11.1

Number of relevant publications in the literature, showing that the majority is in the last decade [3].

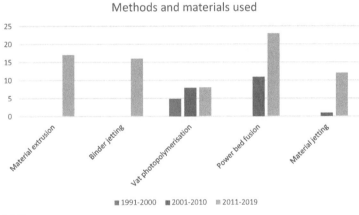

Methods and materials used

■ 1991-2000   ■ 2001-2010   ■ 2011-2019

FIGURE 11.2

Variation of methodologies and materials used throughout the years [3].

dissection. Rhinology-related studies were fewer, and most of them had to do with surgical training. The same review article also demonstrated the chronological distribution of the relevant publications and also the different printing methodologies (Figs. 11.1 and 11.2) [3].

Education and training

Several studies have explored the use of 3D printing technologies in medical education and more specifically in surgical training. Significant advantages are patient safety, favorable supervision in a less stressful environment, no need for cadaveric dissection equipment most of the times, cadaveric specimens can be saved, and the surgical procedures can be standardized and reproduced. An additional advantage is the haptic feedback that is more realistic compared to virtual reality applications. The availability of 3D printing equipment has increased over the past several years, and the cost is getting more affordable.

According to Canzi et al. (2018), there are 23 studies in the literature focusing on otologic applications in training, mainly having to do with temporal bone surgery simulation [3]. In 2015, a temporal bone model based on CT scan data of two selected patients was developed, with well-pneumatized and disease-free mastoids. The final evaluation of the models showed satisfactory reproducibility of most structures and anatomical landmarks but also raised two major issues: the accuracy of the ossicular chain (mainly the stapes) and also the retained resin within the mastoid air cells. The latter impacts on the drilling experience and can be overcome by adding a small drain hole in the region of the sigmoid sinus. The authors concluded that the model produced is useful for training, without depleting a limited supply of cadavers and by using conventional (nonsurgical) tools, such as Dremel drill [7]. On the other hand, it is still difficult to approach the "natural" structure of the cadaveric specimen, mainly due to the "stair stepping" artifact and the lack of anatomical elements such as the dura, nerves, blood vessels, tympanic membrane, and oval and round windows [8].

Another study by Rose et al. (2015) demonstrated satisfactory reproducibility of pediatric temporal bone models. This was confirmed by the measurements of three basic distances on the printed model, CT scan and patient during surgery: 1) sigmoid to posterior canal wall, 2) sigmoid to anterior canal wall, and 3) height of bony external auditory canal. The results demonstrated significant anatomic detail and accuracy [9].

Other groups also confirmed the similarity to the cadaveric specimens and the positive feedback from the trainees [10−12]. More specifically, Hochman et al. (2014) showed that the tactile feedback is satisfactory by analyzing subjective and objective methods. The improvement of materials has provided a better simulation of bone consistency, resulting in a more realistic experience [13]. A useful adjunct in training is the coupling with electronic simulators which offers the possibility of real-time alert in case of vital structural injury. An example is the ElePhant model (Electronic Phantom), where the facial nerve is replaced with a conductive alloy or fiberoptic material, allowing immediate feedback [14].

There are fewer publications on the applications of 3D printing in the field of Rhinology. The main topic addressed in these publications is medium- to high-fidelity simulators of the paranasal sinuses and anterior skull base anatomy, giving the opportunity to trainees to practice drilling via an endonasal approach. It is important to highlight that complex sinonasal and anterior skull procedures are carried out at tertiary, dedicated centers; thus, some trainees may rarely have the opportunity to attend or participate [15−17]. Another useful application was introduced by Chiesa. Estomba et al. (2016) who printed a 3D model for epistaxis management training, combined with a hydraulic system. This permitted residents to practice on the management of anterior and posterior epistaxis, as the model simulated the anterior and posterior ethmoidal arteries, sphenopalatine artery, and Little's area [18].

Finally, interesting applications have been introduced in order to simulate trans-cervical injection of vocal cords [19], bronchoscopy on a 3D printed tracheobron-chial tree [20], various pediatric laryngeal abnormalities such as subglottic cysts, laryngomalacia, subglottic stenosis, and laryngeal clefts [21], and balloon dilatation on 3D-printed cricoid cartilage models [22].

The role of 3D printing in training is very promising in the near future, as new materials and technologically advanced printers will provide greater precision and significant similarity to real anatomy. Moreover, models can be printed with specific pathologies, which can help in preparation prior to surgery or training on more com-plex and rare pathologies, which the average trainee may never encounter.

Surgical planning and patient education

3D printing has significantly contributed to better doctor-patient communication, un-derstanding of the anatomy and comprehension of the disease state and proposed treatment. Sander et al. (2017) introduced a multimaterial sinus model based on clin-ical imaging data, which helped patients understand their treatment plan and improve medical outcomes [23]. The challenging design of osteoplastic flaps can be facilitated by 3D-printed cutting guides [24], and complex sinonasal pathologies can be printed in order to allow preoperative practice, ensuring safer surgery and reduced surgical time. Several publications describe the benefits of 3D-printed models in preoperative planning in otology, cochlear implantation, rhinoplasty, facial plastics, laryngeal framework/tracheal cases, and reconstruction surgery [1,3,25].

Tissue engineering and prosthetics

Several publications have demonstrated the valuable contribution of 3D printing in clinical situations and the progress that has been made so far is promising for future applications.

3D-printed biocompatible scaffolds can work as a framework for chondrocyte aggregation with promising applications in tracheal reconstruction. Such studies have been carried out in vitro and in rabbits, with encouraging results [26–29].

Esophageal patches have been printed and assessed on rabbits, promising easier reconstruction techniques compared to gastric pull-up [30]. In the same direction, Javia et al. (2012) demonstrated that external 3D-printed splint can be used in treat-ing tracheomalacia during upper airway reconstruction [31]. The use of 3D-printed external splint was also studied by Gorostidi et al. (2016) [32].

In the field of Rhinology and facial plastics, there have been efforts to fabricate artificial alar cartilage made of gum resin [33], customized septal buttons for the treatment of septal perforations which provide superior compliance and effectiveness [34]. Also, 3D printing methods have contributed to auricular reconstruction [35].

Studies on tympanic membrane printing, with superior resistance compared to temporalis fascia [36] and superior semicircular canal dehiscence repair with customized prostheses [37] have been published.

Finally, some applications of 3D printing have been explored in the field of Head and Neck surgery, mainly having to do with reconstruction. More specifically, several studies have presented the benefits of 3D printing in mandibular reconstruction, plates, meshes, and mandibular implants. They report good aesthetic and functional outcomes [3].

Future perspectives

At present, the progress in technology and materials has lowered the cost of 3D printing significantly. In addition, collaboration between scientists has given the opportunity for free exchange of models in .STL form (National Institutes of Health's 3D Print Exchange) (3dprint.nih.gov) [38].

Based on the existing literature (which is growing exponentially), there is still room for improvement when it comes to model accuracy and material tactile feedback. Materials which resemble the bone and soft tissues more closely will allow better simulation and consequently achieve one of the basic aims of 3D printing in education, which is surgical training, and hopefully replace cadaveric specimens in the surgical training laboratory. Moreover, there has been progress in bioprinting, and this is a key area in the future of 3D printing in Otolaryngology. Osseous and cartilaginous grafts can replace missing or diseased tissues with low rejection risk; plates and meshes can be designed to fit exactly the recipient areas, leading to accuracy and decreased surgical times. Tracheal bioprinted grafts and stents will revolutionize tracheal reconstruction surgery. It may be possible in the near future to use functional 3D-printed grafts for reconstruction, to the patient's benefit.

References

[1] Crafts TD, Ellsperman SE, Wannemuehler TJ, Bellicchi TD, Shipchandler TZ, Mantravadi AV. Three-dimensional printing and its applications in otorhinolaryngology–head and neck surgery. Otolaryngol Neck Surg 2017;156(6):999–1010.

[2] Gross BC, Erkal JL, Lockwood SY, Chen C, Spence DM. Evaluation of 3D printing and its potential impact on biotechnology and the chemical sciences. ACS Publications; 2014.

[3] Canzi P, Magnetto M, Marconi S, Morbini P, Mauramati S, Aprile F, et al. New frontiers and emerging applications of 3D printing in ENT surgery: a systematic review of the literature. Acta Otorhinolaryngol Ital 2018;38(4):286.

[4] Hull CW. Apparatus for production of three-dimensional objects by stereolithography. Google Patents; 1986.

[5]   Auricchio F, Marconi S. 3D printing: clinical applications in orthopaedics and traumatology. EFORT open Rev 2016;1(5):121−7.

[6]   No title. Comm F42 addit manuf technol [internet]. Available from: www.astm.org/COMMITTEE/F42.html.

[7]   Yushkevich PA, Piven J, Hazlett HC, Smith RG, Ho S, Gee JC, et al. User-guided 3D active contour segmentation of anatomical structures: significantly improved efficiency and reliability. Neuroimage 2006;31(3):1116−28.

[8]   Cohen J, Reyes SA. Creation of a 3D printed temporal bone model from clinical CT data. Am J Otolaryngol 2015;36(5):619−24.

[9]   Rose AS, Webster CE, Harrysson OLA, Formeister EJ, Rawal RB, Iseli CE. Pre-operative simulation of pediatric mastoid surgery with 3D-printed temporal bone models. Int J Pediatr Otorhinolaryngol 2015;79(5):740−4.

[10] Da Cruz MJ, Francis HW. Face and content validation of a novel three-dimensional printed temporal bone for surgical skills development. J Laryngol Otol 2015;129(S3):S23−9.

[11] Hochman JB, Rhodes C, Wong D, Kraut J, Pisa J, Unger B. Comparison of cadaveric and isomorphic three-dimensional printed models in temporal bone education. Laryngoscope 2015;125(10):2353−7.

[12] Mowry SE, Jammal H, Myer IVC, Solares CA, Weinberger P. A novel temporal bone simulation model using 3D printing techniques. Otol Neurotol 2015;36(9):1562−5.

[13] Hochman JB, Kraut J, Kazmerik K, Unger BJ. Generation of a 3D printed temporal bone model with internal fidelity and validation of the mechanical construct. Otolaryngol Neck Surg 2014;150(3):448−54.

[14] Grunert R, Strauss G, Moeckel H, Hofer M, Poessneck A, Fickweiler U, et al. Elephant-an anatomical electronic phantom as simulation-system for otologic surgery. In: Engineering in medicine and biology society, 2006 EMBS'06 28th annual international conference of the IEEE; 2006. p. 4408−11.

[15] Tai BL, Wang AC, Joseph JR, Wang PI, Sullivan SE, McKean EL, et al. A physical simulator for endoscopic endonasal drilling techniques. J Neurosurg 2016;124(3):811−6.

[16] Narayanan V, Narayanan P, Rajagopalan R, Karuppiah R, Rahman ZAA, Wormald P-J, et al. Endoscopic skull base training using 3D printed models with pre-existing pathology. Eur Arch Oto-Rhino-Laryngology 2015;272(3):753−7.

[17] Chan HHL, Siewerdsen JH, Vescan A, Daly MJ, Prisman E, Irish JC. 3D rapid prototyping for otolaryngology—head and neck surgery: applications in image-guidance, surgical simulation and patient-specific modeling. PLoS One 2015;10(9):e0136370.

[18] Chiesa CME, González IF, Iglesias MÁO. How we do it: anterior and posterior nose bleed trainer, the 3D printing epistaxis project. Clin Otolaryngol 2016.

[19] Ainsworth TA, Kobler JB, Loan GJ, Burns JA. Simulation model for transcervical laryngeal injection providing real-time feedback. Ann Otol Rhinol Laryngol 2014;123(12):881−6.

[20] Bustamante S, Bose S, Bishop P, Klatte R, Norris F. Novel application of rapid prototyping for simulation of bronchoscopic anatomy. J Cardiothorac Vasc Anesth 2014;28(4):1122−5.

[21] Kavanagh KR, Cote V, Tsui Y, Kudernatsch S, Peterson DR, Valdez TA. Pediatric laryngeal simulator using 3D printed models: a novel technique. Laryngoscope 2017;127(4):E132−7.

[22] Johnson CM, Howell JT, Mettenburg DJ, Rueggeberg FA, Howell RJ, Postma GN, et al. Mechanical modeling of the human cricoid cartilage using computer-aided design:

applications in airway balloon dilation research. Ann Otol Rhinol Laryngol 2016; 125(1):69−76.

[23] Sander IM, Liepert TT, Doney EL, Leevy WM, Liepert DR. Patient education for endoscopic sinus surgery: preliminary experience using 3D-printed clinical imaging data. J Funct Biomater 2017;8(2):13.

[24] Daniel M, Watson J, Hoskison E, Sama A. Frontal sinus models and onlay templates in osteoplastic flap surgery. J Laryngol Otol 2011;125(1):82−5.

[25] Zhong N, Zhao X. 3D printing for clinical application in otorhinolaryngology. Eur Arch Oto-Rhino-Laryngology 2017;274(12):4079−89.

[26] Goldstein TA, Smith BD, Zeltsman D, Grande D, Smith LP. Introducing a 3-dimensionally printed, tissue-engineered graft for airway reconstruction: a pilot study. Otolaryngol Neck Surg 2015;153(6):1001−6.

[27] Park JH, Park JY, Nam I-C, Hwang S-H, Kim C-S, Jung JW, et al. Human turbinate mesenchymal stromal cell sheets with bellows graft for rapid tracheal epithelial regeneration. Acta Biomater 2015;25:56−64.

[28] Chang JW, Park SA, Park J-K, Choi JW, Kim Y-S, Shin YS, et al. Tissue-engineered tracheal reconstruction using three-dimensionally printed artificial tracheal graft: preliminary report. Artif Organs 2014;38(6):E95−105.

[29] Park JH, Hong JM, Ju YM, Jung JW, Kang H-W, Lee SJ, et al. A novel tissue-engineered trachea with a mechanical behavior similar to native trachea. Biomaterials 2015;62:106−15.

[30] Park SY, Choi JW, Park J-K, Song EH, Park SA, Kim YS, et al. Tissue-engineered artificial oesophagus patch using three-dimensionally printed polycaprolactone with mesenchymal stem cells: a preliminary report. Interact Cardiovasc Thorac Surg 2016; 22(6):712−7.

[31] Javia LR, Zur KB. Laryngotracheal reconstruction with resorbable microplate buttressing. Laryngoscope 2012;122(4):920−4.

[32] Gorostidi F, Reinhard A, Monnier P, Sandu K. External bioresorbable airway rigidification to treat refractory localized tracheomalacia. Laryngoscope 2016;126(11):2605−10.

[33] Xu Y, Fan F, Kang N, Wang S, You J, Wang H, et al. Tissue engineering of human nasal alar cartilage precisely by using three-dimensional printing. Plast Reconstr Surg 2015; 135(2):451−8.

[34] Altunay ZO, Bly JA, Edwards PK, Holmes DR, Hamilton GS, O'Brien EK, et al. Three-dimensional printing of large nasal septal perforations for optimal prosthetic closure. Am J Rhinol Allergy 2016;30(4):287−93.

[35] Bos EJ, Scholten T, Song Y, Verlinden JC, Wolff J, Forouzanfar T, et al. Developing a parametric ear model for auricular reconstruction: a new step towards patient-specific implants. J Cranio-Maxillofacial Surg 2015;43(3):390−5.

[36] Kozin ED, Black NL, Cheng JT, Cotler MJ, McKenna MJ, Lee DJ, et al. Design, fabrication, and in vitro testing of novel three-dimensionally printed tympanic membrane grafts. Hear Res 2016;340:191−203.

[37] Kozin ED, Remenschneider AK, Cheng S, Nakajima HH, Lee DJ. Three-dimensional printed prosthesis for repair of superior canal dehiscence. Otolaryngol Neck Surg 2015;153(4):616−9.

[38] Ventola CL. Medical applications for 3D printing: current and projected uses. Pharm Ther 2014;39(10):704.

[39] Bandyopadhyay A, Bose S, Das S. 3D printing of biomaterials. MRS Bull 2015;40(2): 108−15.

Challenges, opportunities, and limitations in 3D printing

12

Vassilios Tsioukas, PhD [1]**, Christos Pikridas, PhD** [2]**, Ion-Anastasios Karolos, PhD** [3]

[1]*Electrical Engineer, Professor, School of Rural and Surveying Engineering, Aristotle University of Thessaloniki, Thessaloniki, Greece;* [2]*Professor, Rural and Surveying Engineer, School of Rural and Surveying Engineering, Department of Geodesy and Surveying, Aristotle University of Thessaloniki, Thessaloniki, Greece;* [3]*Rural and Surveying Engineer, School of Rural and Surveying Engineering, Aristotle University of Thessaloniki, Thessaloniki, Greece*

Computer-aided design—cost production

More specifically, the pre- and postprinting cost amount to a significant proportion of total cost per printed part. So, even when the cost for printer materials decreases, the labor-cost penalty will remain. A "simple" rule says that if no computer-aided design (CAD) exists, then no 3D print could be done. Getting a CAD is challenging and may require several man-hours in order to produce basic results. It requires persistence and discipline to develop the necessary skill. Therefore, there are many 3D model libraries on the internet for e.g., GrabCAD, Pinshape, Thingiverse, and several others. But here (until today), you can only 3D print what you can find on the sites and with many more limitations existing regarding medical applications.

Types of materials—strength-printing techniques

There is a limited set of materials to print. Most of them are thermoplastics. The ability to print in only a few materials is a major setback in the FDM 3D printing industry. However, plastic may vary in strength capacity and may not be the best for some components. Popular and low-cost 3D printers use a plastic filament. The "first" selection is the biodegradable polylactic acid (PLA), but the ABS (acrylonitrile butadiene styrene) filament is still the most commonly used type of plastic. Some companies offer metal as a material, but final product parts are often not fully dense. Other materials like glass, carbon fiber, and nylon are being used, but have yet to enter commercial production.

Summarizing the current printing technologies, these are found to FDM, SLA, SLS and Polyjet. A fifth CLIP is still currently not as widespread as these four.

Stereolithography or SLA is one of the older and more widely used 3D printing technologies. SLA has a smooth surface finish and allows for fine detail. SLA is limited in terms of materials though, and despite increasing progress on this front, the ones available are still pretty far from production materials. The parts are generally quite brittle and will discolor over time. They are also susceptible to damage by moisture, heat, and chemicals. These specifications, limit the potential applications of parts made by SLA, which means that for the most part it is only useful for prototypes and models.

Selective laser sintering or SLS is a great choice for functional models and even production parts. Their materials are tough and durable. That said, you are again confronted with a lack of choice with SLS; the nylon PA materials are essentially all you have. The powder sintering process also means fine details are difficult to realize via SLS. The parts are porous and have a rough surface which is difficult to polish and paint (though not impossible).

Polyjet is a Stratasys technology (https://www.stratasys.com/) that shoots very thin layers of liquid photopolymer to build complex, detailed parts with smooth surfaces. Polyjet also allows you to combine multiple colors and materials in one print so you can create overmolded parts or detailed display models. Despite the multiple material choices available, they all remain of the same ilk and as such are limited in terms of the properties, and like SLA materials not very durable. The build accuracy is different in different directions, and due to the layered build process, there is also a stepping effect on some surfaces.

We have presented above the basics of the technology specific limitations and there is also one major limitation facing all current 3D printing processes—the build size. This is also a critical factor in medical surgery. All of these technologies are limited by the size of the machines, and the larger they get, the more issues you have with accuracy across the whole build table. It is possible to split and glue parts produced from FDM or SLA, for example, but again you are losing strength and accuracy. Compact printing objects may more easily produced by the metal 3D printing. This will probably only pay off as a substitute for casting at the earliest by 2020, metal printers are already profitable for small batch sizes. This is because molding is still much cheaper.

Customer satisfaction—after market services

The 3D-printed part when taken out of the 3D printer usually has a bad-to-mediocre surface finish. Postprocessing techniques like sanding, acetone treatment, or putty treatment are necessary for a smooth surface finish on the part.

In all the major 3D printers, you cannot 3D print in more than one color. To make a colored item using a 3D printer, you will first have to 3D print it in white and then paint it, and painting is not easy, unless done by a professional of course.

Challenges in 3D printing

3D printing, also known as additive manufacturing, is based on the principle of layered manufacturing, in which materials are overlapped layer by layer using fast and reasonably priced equipment. Current challenges of research on 3D printing technology for medical applications in general can be classified into the following areas.

Organ models

The use of 3D models within the medical profession has been around since the dissection of human cadavers in ancient Greece. With the help of 3D printing, synthetic modeling of organs and human anatomy has made a significant step forward. Human cadavers from ancient days have given way to synthetic models with the look and feel of human tissue. Eventual reproduction and regeneration of tissue are now much closer to reality. Recent advancements in 3D printing technologies have facilitated the creation of patient-specific organ models with the purpose of providing an effective solution for preoperative planning, rehearsal, and spatiotemporal mapping.

Prosthetic parts—personalized plaster (proplasma)

Because of the complexity of making a prosthetic part, the SLA desktop 3D printing has been found as the most accurate, durable, and cost-effective parts for this job. Using a combination of plastics, 3D printers fabricate modular prosthetics tailored to a patient's anatomy and needs. Prosthetics should be designed to fit individuals' unique needs and preferences, just like in contraception. There is also the time and financial cost to patients, who (in many cases) have to travel long distances for treatment that can take several days in order to assess their need, produce a prosthesis, and fit it to the residual limb. The result is that braces and artificial limbs are among the most desperately needed medical devices. The first person to test out a 3D-printed mobility device was a four-year-old girl. For the case of artificial fingers, the prosthetic procedure begins by creating a CAD template, as is always the case with the 3D technology. The printed parts are primarily made from PLA or ABS material and are used to create the major structure, such as the palms and fingers.

3D printing biomaterials

Bioprinting is a term that has been referring to 3D printing actual living organs and tissues. In this process, the first step is to take a biopsy of the organ or tissue to be replaced. Among different types of 3D printing techniques, extrusion-based and inkjet-based 3D printing methods are commonly used for bioprinting. Due to the nature of 3D printing methods, most of the ceramics materials are combined with polymers to enhance their printability. Polymer-based biomaterials are 3D printed mostly using extrusion-based printing and have a wide range of applications in regenerative medicine. Naturally occurring biomaterials, such as collagen, chitosan, hyaluronic acid, alginate, etc., are widely used because of their biodegradability, biocompatibility, and abundant availability. Important factors to make biomaterials suitable for 3D printing processes are rheological properties and the method of cross-linking. Various mixtures for producing bio-based material products are possible. For example, scientists proposed that it is possible to blend bio-based plastics with other bio-base plastics, such as TPS with PLA. But it is also common to blend bio-based plastics with fossil-based plastics, for example, PLA with PBAT. This blend still has its biodegradable functionality, as both the bio-based PLA and the fossil-based PBAT are compostable. Blending is another way and is applied tailor-made for a wide range of applications.

Generally, speaking bioprinting can be defined as additive three-dimensional fabrication of tissues or organs using cells, biomaterials, and biological molecules. Until today, three main categories could be found in bioprinting.

- Jet-based bioprinting, which is a noncontact technique in which 2D and 3D structures are generated using picoliter bioink droplets layered onto a substrate.
- Extrusion-based bioprinting, which dispenses continuous filaments of a material consisting of cells mixed with hydrogel through a micronozzle to fabricate 2D or 3D structures.
- Integrated bioprinting, which is the well-known bioprinting technology and relies on cell-laden hydrogels and cell aggregates to fabricate structures.

Opportunities in 3D printing

General speaking, the flexibility of 3D printing allows designers to make changes easily without the need to set up additional equipment or tools. These capabilities have sparked huge interest in 3D printing of medical devices. More specific, major attractions in the growth of the global market of 3D printing are the dental applications.

Printable dental products are classified as medical devices, and they can have the following uses: replace or repair a damaged tooth, create an orthodontic model, produce crowns, bridges, caps, and dentures, and construct surgical tools.

3D printing technology is going to transform medicine, whether it is patient-specific surgical models, custom-made prosthetics, personalized on-demand medicines, or even 3D-printed human tissue. As its core 3D printing is the use of computer guidance technology to create 3D objects, medicine is just another frontier and challenge. Based on the available literature, 3D printing is on the way to making this possible, opening up a whole new world of customized medicines. As a consequence, maybe that in the near future instead of a prescription, your doctor will be giving you a digital file of printing instructions.

By utilizing the cloud-based technology, there will be a delivery concept of CAD and modeling software from teaching hospitals and specialty centers into the broader hospital system. Right now, only a small number of hospitals and research institutions have 3D printing capabilities on site, according to the report. But as more 3D printing capabilities come online, increased demand for 3D printing from the medical staff can be expected. In the future, in-house 3D printers could possibly be used in hospitals to rapidly churn out body parts not only for practice, but also to meet the needs of emergency trauma patients.

According to international conference proceedings on 3D printing in Medicine, printing technology has a significant role in regenerative medicine. Using the 3D printing process, veins, nerves, breast tissue, bone replacement material, or corneas can already be artificially produced today. Bioprinting technology, which supports the reproduction of organic tissue, enables the precise arrangement of living, human cells in three-dimensional structures. It is seen as a key technology for producing functional tissue or whole organs in future. This synergy is also intended to combine synergies among participants from different areas, to work out and support any national and international cooperation projects.

Nevertheless, it seems the applications for 3D printing are endless. Scientists have churned out everything from houses to rocket parts, blood vessels to artificial limbs. Now, to add to the ever-growing collection of awesome 3D-printed goodies, medics have used the famous additive manufacturing technology to produce replicas of infants' brains in order to practice life-saving but risky surgical procedures. Having a detailed model of the brain to work with means that surgeons are no longer reliant on MRI scans and instinct to perform highly complex and precise operations.

Further reading

[1]   Kalaskar DM. 3D printing in medicine. Woodhead publishing; 2017.
[2]   Noorani R. 3D printing.technology, applications, and selection. CRC Press; 2018.

Index

Printed and bound by CPI Group (UK) Ltd, Croydon, CR0 4YY

03/10/2024

01040300-0017